Natural WEIGHT LOSS Miracles

Natural WEIGHT LOSS Miracles

20 Wonder Pills, Powders, and Supplements
to Burn Fat and Shed Pounds Naturally

Maggie Greenwood-Robinson, Ph.D.

A Perigee Book

The suggestions for specific supplements, foods, and exercise are not intended to replace medical advice or treatment by your physician. All questions and concerns regarding your health, weight, and physical activity should be directed to your physician, particularly if you have any health problems or medical problems, (including if you are pregnant or breast-feeding). Long-term use of a nutritional supplementation is not recommended unless it is done under the guidance and supervision of a physician.

All reasonable attempts have been made to include the most recent and factual research and medical reports about natural weight-loss supplements. However, there is no guarantee that future research, particularly human studies, will not change the recommendations and information presented here. Individual needs vary, and no supplement, diet, or exercise plan will meet everyone's daily needs. Be sure to consult your physician prior to following any of the suggestions in this book.

The mention of specific products or brands in this book does not constitute an endorsement by either the author or the publisher.

A Perigee Book
Published by The Berkley Publishing Group
A member of Penguin Putnam Inc.
375 Hudson Street
New York, New York 10014

First edition: March 1999

Published simultaneously in Canada.

The Penguin Putnam Inc. World Wide Web site address is
http://www.penguinputnam.com

Library of Congress Cataloging-in-Publication Data

Greenwood-Robinson, Maggie.
    Natural weight loss miracles : 20 wonder pills, powders, and
supplements to burn fat and shed pounds naturally / Maggie Greenwood-
Robinson.
      p.   cm.
    "A Perigee book."
    Includes bibliographical references.
    ISBN 0-399-52479-7
    1. Weight loss. 2. Naturopathy. 3. Dietary supplements.
    4. Herbs—Therapeutic use. I. Title.
    RM222.2.G725   1999
    613.2—dc21   98-43495
                                               CIP

Printed in the United States of America

10 9 8 7 6 5 4 3 2 1

To my nieces Erin Grace Greenwood and Taylor Joan Ortiz

CONTENTS

ACKNOWLEDGMENTS

Natural Weight Loss Miracles has become a reality due to the energy and efforts of the following people:

Claire Gerus, my agent who is an experienced, tireless professional in her field, a crusader for sound natural health practices, and a true believer in my work;

Sheila Curry and the staff of Perigee Books, my very first publisher, with whom I started more than 10 years ago and who gave me the opportunity to put this very important information in print;

My husband, Jeff, who has encouraged me in my career and has given me the love and inspiration to persevere.

— *Maggie Greenwood-Robinson, Ph.D.*

Natural WEIGHT LOSS Miracles

LOSING WEIGHT THE NATURAL WAY

It's a dieter's dream: a magic pill that melts fat, and with no side effects.

Good news: Scientists are closer than ever to making that dream come true. New research into obesity has unraveled many mysteries about why we eat and how we store and burn off calories. As a result, pharmaceutical companies are spending extraordinary sums to develop new generations of anti-obesity drugs, and many are now in test phases.

In the meantime, we're fighting fat, often unsuccessfully, and spending about $30 billion a year to do so. How long do we have to wait for that "magic pill"?

Actually, we don't have to wait. On the shelves of pharmacies and health food stores are nutritional supplements that can help end your weight-loss struggles for good. These natural weight-loss agents are effective, easily obtainable, and safe for most people. They don't even require a prescription.

While not magical per se, many natural weight-loss products can bring miraculous results when it comes to fat loss and weight control, such as tweaking your body's metabolism for faster fat-burning, suppressing your appetite naturally, energizing your body, and more.

To understand why the natural weight-loss supplements offer so much promise, it's helpful to review a little history regarding diet pills.

DIET PILLS—A TROUBLING PAST

The quest to find a slimming pill has been ongoing and never-ending. Every generation has had its version. In the 1930s, bath salts and orange pekoe tea were pitched as cures for obesity. The 1950s brought laxatives and mineral preparations promising to erase flabby bulges. In the 1960s and 1970s, doctors prescribed amphetamines (also known as "speed"), which incinerated calories by jump-starting the body's metabolism. But they were also addictive, and diet pills got a bad name as a result.

In 1996, the Food and Drug Administration (FDA) approved a new anti-obesity drug, dexfenfluramine, sold under the brand name Redux. It worked by triggering the release of serotonin, a brain chemical that when elevated makes you feel full. Dexfenfluramine joined two other appetite-suppressing drugs already on the market, phentermine and fenfluramine. Like dexfenfluramine, fenfluramine caused the brain to release more serotonin, suppressing the appetite. Phentermine, on the other hand, jacked up the nervous system and quashed the appetite much as amphetamines did but without being addictive. Known popularly as "phen-fen," phentermine and fenfluramine were used in tandem to produce a powerful appetite-curbing effect.

All three drugs were meant primarily for people who were considered obese, defined as being 20 percent or more above ideal weight. But abuses were rampant. Some physicians prescribed them for women who wanted to drop just a dress size, or who wanted to shed only a few pounds.

The drugs have disturbing side effects. Fenfluramine can cause dry mouth, drowsiness, diarrhea, and, less frequently, heart palpitations. Phentermine can produce dry mouth, too, as well as nervousness, constipation, and insomnia. Dexfenfluramine has a rare but potentially fatal side effect—primary pulmonary hypertension, in which the blood vessels supplying the lungs become scarred and thickened. The disease is progressive, ending in death within a few years.

Furthermore, evidence surfaced that the drugs didn't work as well as promised. A Cornell University nutrition professor reviewed all the available studies on fenfluramine and dexfenfluramine and found that dieters taking the drugs lost only an average of 5 pounds, often the same amount shed with a placebo. Not a very impressive track record.

Nonetheless, physicians wrote an average of 85,000 prescriptions a week for dexfenfluramine alone. And many commercial weight-loss centers jumped on the bandwagon, handing out prescriptions for the drugs without the written consent or knowledge of the dieter's own doctor.

Then, in September 1997, newspapers around the country had shocking news for dieters: Fenfluramine and dexfenfluramine were yanked from the market after a Mayo Clinic study found that 30 percent of 290 patients who took them showed signs of heart-valve abnormalities. Later, the FDA estimated that one-third of people taking these pills could have suffered heart-valve damage. Dieters who had taken these drugs were urged to see their physicians for a complete heart-valve checkup. By the end of 1997, the FDA had begun investigating whether phen-fen and dexfenfluramine could be implicated in birth defects.

Controversy over the drugs still simmers. A large study conducted at

Georgetown University, released in April 1998, found no evidence that dexfenfluramine caused heart-valve problems during the two or three months dieters usually took it. However, the study did suggest that long-term use of the drug could pose dangers.

In 1998, a new weight-loss drug, sibutramine (Meridia), received a thumbs-up from the FDA, even over the objections of its own scientific advisers. It is designed to treat serious obesity, especially cases accompanied by other health problems, such as diabetes.

Sibutramine works differently from other prescription weight-loss drugs. It doesn't boost levels of serotonin, but prevents it from being reabsorbed. This helps keep levels high, creating a sensation of fullness. The drug also raises levels of another brain chemical, noradrenaline (also known as norepinephrine), to help stimulate the metabolism. Research shows that sibutramine promotes weight loss of 5 to 10 percent—not as much as people lost while taking phen fen. Like most weight-loss agents, sibutramine is most beneficial when used with proper diet and exercise.

But doubts about the safety of sibutramine linger. Side effects include dry mouth, headache, constipation, and insomnia. More serious side effects include increases in blood pressure and pulse rate—both of which could be life-threatening to people with hypertension or certain heart conditions. Time will tell whether the drug will work effectively or go the way of its predecessors.

Another drug on the horizon is orlistat (Xenical), which blocks intestinal enzymes from absorbing 30 percent of fat that is eaten. The fat is excreted without being stored. Interestingly, there are a couple of natural weight-loss substances that do the very same thing—bind with fat and help carry it out of the body.

Other prescription drugs are either in the pipeline or close to approval. In table 1.1 (page 14), you'll find a list of currently available drugs, those possibly coming soon, and natural, supplemental alternatives to each one.

SAFER ALTERNATIVES

In the wake of the ongoing concern over the safety of prescription diet pills, the weight-conscious public is asking: Now what?

The answer: natural weight-loss supplements!

When taken properly, these nutritional agents carry none of the risks of prescription diet pills. Most of these products are simply nutrients, extracted from food or plants. While producing weight loss, they have a much gentler effect on your body than prescription medications have. You should consider using natural weight-loss supplements if:

· You need to lose ten pounds or more.

· You want to suppress your appetite and curb cravings naturally.

· You don't want to expose your body to the potentially health-damaging effects of prescription weight-loss drugs.

· You've given up on prescription weight-loss drugs and are seeking a safer solution.

· You need temporary and safe weight-loss assistance while trying to change your eating habits permanently.

You really have nothing to lose, except unsightly fat, by taking a more natural approach to weight loss. In fact, you have everything to gain in terms of better health, more energy, and an improved self-image!

You may be wondering: Are these products safe? Good question! Unlike prescription medicines, nutritional supplements aren't approved by the FDA. Under the Dietary Supplement Health and Education Act of 1994, supplement manufacturers can make nutrition support statements about their products—statements that describe how the product functions in the body. But they aren't allowed to claim that the product can treat or cure any disease. Also, supplement labels must carry the following disclaimer: "This statement has not been evaluated by the Food and Drug Administration. This product is not intended to diagnose, treat, cure, or prevent any disease."

But just because natural weight-loss supplements and other nutritional supplements aren't approved by the FDA, that doesn't mean they're unsafe. Over the years, there have been many pharmaceutical agents that won FDA approval but due to serious, sometimes fatal, effects were pulled from the market.

Keep in mind that natural weight-loss supplements are derived from food or herbs—and thus work with your body rather than against it (as many prescription medicines do). It's always preferable to try the gentlest agent first. Some of these supplements do have some minor side effects, but they are far less serious than those of prescription diet pills.

Also, there is a wealth of scientific evidence demonstrating the effectiveness of natural weight-loss products—evidence you'll read about here. Plus, many of these supplements have other health-promotion benefits. Natural supplements do many things! That's one of their most redeeming values.

WHY SLIMMER IS BETTER

Natural weight-loss supplements are one more weapon against obesity—a disease that's killing us and draining our pocketbooks. Health experts report that a majority of the world's population is now overweight, and that obesity costs consumers billions of dollars a year for health care. In the United States alone, the financial toll of obesity is more than $100 billion annually.

In fact, the United States has one of the highest rates of obesity in the world. According to a recent survey, nearly 74 percent of Americans age 25 or older are overweight. After smoking, which causes an estimated 500,000 deaths a year, weight-related conditions are the second leading cause of death in the United States, claiming 300,000 lives each year. But other developed countries are not far behind. In 1997, the *British Medical Journal* reported that the prevalence of obesity in many countries is now so high that it should be considered a pandemic—which means an exceptionally large portion of the world is on the pudgy side.

Although overweight and obesity are considered to be appearance problems, they are in fact serious conditions, directly linked to a number of disabling and life-threatening diseases. Among them are heart disease, stroke, some cancers, diabetes, high blood pressure, gall bladder disease, osteoarthritis, and mental health problems.

Why is obesity so deadly? Take the number-one killer, heart disease, for example. Obesity places a strain on the heart. It enlarges the heart's ventricles, alters its function, and leads to other structural abnormalities.

Studies indicate that obese adults aged 20 to 45 are at nearly four times the risk of developing diabetes and more than five times the risk of getting high blood pressure than normal-weight adults.

Obese men have a significantly greater chance of dying from cancer of the colon, rectum, and prostate, and obese women have a greater risk of developing endometrial and postmenopausal breast cancers.

Plump women whose body fat is distributed around and above the waist run a particularly high risk of developing endometrial cancer, one of the most common cancers that afflict women. It usually occurs after menopause, and if detected early, it's almost always curable. Scientists speculate that one reason for the risk is that upper-body-obese women have higher levels of the female hormone estrogen, which can set the stage for endometrial cancer.

Like endometrial cancer, most breast cancers have a hormonal link. As noted above, women with excess upper body fat have higher levels of estrogen, and some investigators think that these women run a significantly higher risk of developing breast cancer. Obesity doesn't cause breast cancer, but it encourages the spread of existing cancer.

If you're obese, your bile may be oversaturated with cholesterol, a blood fat, and this can lead to the formation of gallstones.

Until only recently, it was assumed that a little weight gain at any age was okay. But studies have found that even a tiny gain can increase your odds of having a heart attack. In 1995, the U.S. Department of Agriculture (USDA) published new guidelines that said middle-age spread was unhealthy and that for good health, people in their sixties should weigh the same as trim people in their thirties.

Backing up the USDA's recommendations was one of the largest studies ever to examine the effects of weight on longevity. Published in 1998 in the *New England Journal of Medicine*, the study concluded that slimmer is definitely better at any age, including middle age and beyond.

This conclusion was based on American Cancer Society data on 324,135 men and women enrolled in the study in 1960 and then followed up in 1972. The data revealed that being overweight tended to shorten life expectancy up to about age 75. After that age, being heavy didn't make much of a difference unless someone was seriously obese. People who maintained a healthy, ideal weight generally lived the longest.

THE PROMISE OF NATURAL WEIGHT-LOSS SUPPLEMENTS

Overweight and obesity are caused by multiple factors, and natural weight-loss supplements can tackle many of them. Let's take a closer look.

· **Overeating.** If you habitually eat more calories than you burn off, the surplus is stored as body fat. So why do we overeat? There's no simple explanation, really, but a lot of it has to do with *hunger, appetite,* and *satiety*—mechanisms that tell us when to eat and how much. They are centered in the hypothalamus, a small area of the brain located in the middle of the skull. The hypothalamus is the body's center for controlling food intake. It also regulates thirst, metabolism, and body temperature.

Hunger is largely a physiological drive. About every four hours, your body signals that it's time to eat by creating sensations such as hunger pangs or a feeling of low energy. After you start eating a meal, it takes about twenty minutes for your body to send satiety signals to the hypothalamus that you're full. Continuing to eat beyond that points leaves you feeling stuffed. By eating when you're hungry and stopping when you're full, you'll have little trouble maintaining a healthy weight.

Just recently, it was discovered that the hypothalamus produces a hunger hormone, dubbed "orexin" after *orexis*, the Greek word for hunger. When the brain senses a need to eat, such as after a drop in blood sugar, it starts producing more orexin.

Lots of factors trigger hunger or lack of it: disease, emotions, weather (cold increases hunger, hot decreases it), the composition of your diet (a well-balanced diet keeps hunger pangs in check), to name just a few.

Hunger is different from appetite. The best way to understand the difference is this: With hunger, you eat in response to physical sensations (like hunger pangs). With appetite, you eat in response to cravings for certain foods—cravings based on foods you grew up loving, social situations such as parties or holidays, or mood states such as depression or anxiety. Additionally, you may crave certain foods for physiological reasons. For example, a woman may hanker for chocolate during her period—a craving probably triggered by hormonal fluctuations, since hormones play a role in regulating appetite. Thus, appetite is influenced by many social, cultural, psychological, and physiological factors.

Appetite, like hunger, is controlled by the hypothalamus. In fact, the hypothalamus can switch appetite off and on, in much the way a thermostat regulates room temperature. Appetite and hunger often accompany one another, increasing or decreasing our desire and need for food.

The search for safe and effective appetite-killing drugs continues. Some success has been achieved, but not without great cost to health. Fortunately, though, effective alternatives are available. There are many natural appetite suppressants that appear to curb overeating safely.

- **Undereating.** Believe it or not, chronic calorie-cutting can make you fat! Overly restricting your calories below 1,200 if you're a woman, or below 1,600 if you're a man, can slow your metabolism—the body's food-to-fuel process. This results in something called the "starvation adaptation response." Without adequate calories, your body is tricked into thinking it's starving. As a built-in survival mechanism, a special fat storage enzyme (*lipoprotein lipase*) mounted on the surface of fat cells in the body goes to work, signaling your body to stockpile dietary fat rather than burn it for energy. You can actually gain body fat on a diet of less than 1,200 calories a day, not to mention skimp on important nutrients. That's why it's both unwise and unhealthy to cut calories drastically. Several natural weight-loss supplements let you eat ample calories, without restrictive dieting, and still lose appreciable amounts of body fat.

· **Underexercising.** Are you physically inactive? Being a couch potato is a major contributor to obesity—even more than overeating is, say some health experts. Generally, people are now eating smaller amounts of fattening foods, but paradoxically, obesity is on the rise. Lack of physical activity may be the most reasonable explanation. If you're not exercising, it could be due to lack of energy. Good news: There are a couple of natural weight-loss supplements that may help energize you for exercise.

· **Genetics.** If one of your parents was obese, you have a 60 percent chance of being plump, too; if both were obese, your chances rise to 90 percent. No one knows for sure why this is so, but researchers have discovered a gene in humans that they've dubbed the *ob* gene. This gene manufactures a hormone called leptin. Leptin is secreted by fat tissue and released into the bloodstream. It then travels to the brain. Its job there is to help the body regulate its fat stores by curbing appetite and stimulating metabolism. Scientists speculate that obese people may be "resistant" to the effects of leptin. In other words, their brain cells are unresponsive to leptin in much the same way body cells of diabetics are unresponsive to insulin. Research on a leptin-based drug has produced mixed results. With diet and exercise, some people lost weight, others lost no weight, and some even got fatter. There are, however, several natural weight-loss substances that do a great job of suppressing the appetite and stimulating the metabolism. These may help you, even if it looks like heredity is not on your side.

· **Thermogenesis.** One theory of obesity holds that plump people may have a slower rate of "thermogenesis"—the body's natural ability to generate heat as a result of breaking down food for energy. The body tissue that specializes in converting energy to heat is brown fat, which is located deep within the body and insulates internal organs. By contrast, white fat cells—found in the muscles and under the skin—tend to store energy.

Scientists have theorized that people who have less than a normal amount of brown fat tend to store more white fat. New research points to the fact that fat cells, both brown and white, of obese people generate less heat—which could result in more calories being stored as bulges. Some of the natural weight-loss supplements now on the market are believed to stimulate the thermogenic capability of brown fat and thus burn more stored fat.

· **Environment.** The type of food available to you may affect whether you eat too much and become overweight. You may live in a region of the country where appetizing but high-fat food—and lots of it—is readily available. According to a study released in 1997 by the Coalition for Excess Weight Risk Reduction, residents in certain parts of the United States are fatter than people elsewhere. New Orleans, for example, has the highest obesity level (37.55 percent of the adult population) in the nation, possibly because of the city's traditional high-fat cuisine. Other high-obesity areas include Cleveland with its high-fat heartland foods; Atlanta, known for its Southern-style comfort foods; and Dallas, where frequent dining out is a part of residents' lifestyle.

But of course the opportunity to overeat may be no farther than your refrigerator! Even so, you can use natural weight-loss supplements to curb your appetite and decrease your food intake, no matter where you live.

· **Virus.** The newest—and one of the most startling—findings about the causes of obesity is a virus. In a preliminary study, researchers at the University of Wisconsin-Madison found that 15 percent of obese people carry antibodies to a virus known to cause obesity in animals. The presence of antibodies indicated that the people were exposed to the virus at one time. But how the infection might cause obesity isn't known. The possibility that some cases of obesity may have a viral origin could help explain why obesity is on the rise—and lead to better cures. However, more investigation is needed into the viral causes of obesity.

TEN IMPORTANT POINTS TO CONSIDER

As a consumer interested in taking natural weight-loss supplements, there are several things you must do first:

1. Educate yourself on natural weight-loss supplements and the research, if any, behind them. If a claim is made regarding weight-loss effectiveness, check it out and learn all you can about the product and its ingredients. Reading this book is an excellent first step, since it reviews many of the diet supplements on the market and describes in detail what they can and cannot do. For instance, many herbs promoted for weight loss are actually diuretics that stimulate fluid loss but have no effect on fat loss. Other good information sources include magazine articles, medical journals, your

doctor, or your pharmacist. There is also information on the Internet; however, a lot of "cyber" information is product promotion.

2. Purchase natural weight-loss supplements from well-known, reputable companies.

3. Read the label on any diet supplement you buy. Make sure you know what each ingredient is and what effect it has on the body. Don't buy the supplement until you have learned all you can about its ingredients and its potential side effects. If you're considering an herbal supplement, purchase a "standardized" product. (See the box below, "Buying Standardized Products.")

4. Tell your doctor you are taking a natural diet supplement, especially during an illness or before surgery. If you don't, you're taking the chance that your doctor may unwittingly prescribe something that will interact dangerously with the supplement.

Communicating with your doctor about supplements is sometimes hard to do. But there are ways to overcome this. For example, when asked what medications you're taking, include supplements, as well as any successes you've had with them. Also, report any unusual symptoms or allergic reactions you may experience.

5. Follow the manufacturer's or doctor's suggestion regarding dosage and diet. Also, pay close attention to any warnings or precautions that appear on the supplement label.

6. Supplements may react negatively with foods, alcohol, or drugs, including prescription medications. Check with your doctor to make sure there are no adverse interactions between supplements and medications.

7. As with medicines, regard supplements as potentially harmful to children, and keep those supplements safely out of their sight and reach.

8. Natural weight-loss supplements work best in combination with a healthy, low-fat diet and a regular exercise program. Permanent lifestyle change is still the best way to lose weight. For information on diet and exercise, see appendix A and appendix B.

9. Don't let diet pills and supplements—natural or otherwise—become a long-term crutch. You can fall into the trap of thinking, "If I'm not taking a pill, I won't lose weight," and get psychologically addicted to pill-popping for weight loss. Diet drugs and supplements aren't required for weight loss. But long-term habit change is. You can lose weight without drugs and supplements as long as you set your mind on doing so. The

beauty of natural weight-loss substances is that they can safely help you in the *short term* while you make *long-term* changes in your eating and exercise habits.

10. After you've achieved your weight-loss goals, you no longer need to take natural weight-loss supplements. However, some products may help you during the maintenance phase of your weight-loss effort.

HOW TO USE THIS BOOK

Natural Weight Loss Miracles is your guide to diet supplements now on the market. It explains why they are preferable to potentially dangerous drugs and drug combinations. The information here is based on the most up-to-date research from nutrition science and supplementation. I have also included a few real-life case studies of people who have used certain supplements with great success. Specifically, this book gives you the latest news on the following:

- Which nutrients will boost your metabolism for more efficient fat-burning

- Which substances can curb your appetite—naturally

- Which supplements work best when combined with an exercise program to accelerate fat loss

- Which nutrients can alter brain chemistry safely and naturally to quell cravings and reduce emotion-driven eating binges

- Which natural supplements should be avoided because they may be as dangerous as prescription weight-loss drugs.

I have organized this book into five parts: natural fat-fighters, natural appetite suppressants, natural metabolic boosters, natural herbs for weight management, and natural weight control. In each part are chapters that cover the specifics about various natural weight-loss supplements. Each chapter describes the particular supplement, how it works, the research behind it, dietary recommendations, and safety considerations.

Although many more natural weight-loss supplements are discussed in this book, there are twenty that I feel are beneficial in a weight-control program, based on current research. They are pyruvate, l-carnitine, chromium, lipotropics, chitin (chitosan), konjac root (glucomannan), psyllium, 5-HTP (5 hydroxy-tryptophan), phenylalanine, tyrosine, methionine, glutamine, MCT oil, creatine, hydroxycitric acid (HCA), guggul, conjugated linoleic acid (CLA), ciwujia, beta-hydroxy beta-methylbutyrate (HMB), and meal replacers.

I have also included three appendices. Appendix A outlines a 21-day eating plan that works well with most natural weight-loss supplements while providing excellent nutrition for dieters. The plan tells you exactly what to eat each day of the week; there's no guesswork involved.

In appendix B, you'll find some tips for exercise, specifically how to fit it into your lifestyle and how to maximize its fat-burning power.

Finally, appendix C provides a lengthy though partial list of the major natural weight-loss products on the market. I've listed the ingredients of each one, so you can see what you're buying and taking. Prices are included, too. Appendix C is a handy reference to consult before you go to your health food store or pharmacy.

This book is not intended to substitute for medical advice or treatment recommended by your physician. If you have concerns about your weight, or suffer from a preexisting illness or medical condition, consult with your doctor before following any of the suggestions in this book or taking any of the supplements.

In this book, you'll find a star rating system for natural weight-loss supplements, showing—at a glance—which ones offer the best potential for fat-loss, are backed by ample research, provide additional health-building benefits, and have the fewest side effects.

★★★★★ The supplement is effective for weight loss, has been extensively studied (in both animals and humans), has many other potential health benefits, and causes very few side effects.

★★★★ The supplement has been shown in numerous studies to be effective for weight loss, offers several health benefits, and causes minimal side effects.

★★★ The supplement has a specific role in weight control (i.e., appetite suppression or enhancement of energy-producing processes) that is backed up by preliminary research. It offers some additional health benefits, and side effects are minimal.

★★ The supplement may support the body's metabolism and have some fat-loss benefit, but research is less extensive. While not directly involved in weight loss, this supplement may play a supporting role in weight management. There may be some side effects.

★ The supplement, while not extensively researched, shows promise. A single star may also indicate that there are more side effects compared with other supplements.

You can use this book as a handbook—an encyclopedia of sorts in which you can skip around and look up chapters that interest you—or you can ready it sequentially, from cover to cover. No matter what course you take, you should have enough information to make informed decisions about which supplements are best for you and your health.

I hope you will use this book to make permanent lifestyle changes in your diet and exercise habits—and ultimately become fit, active, and healthy for the rest of your life.

Table 1-1. Prescription Weight-Loss Drugs and Their Natural Counterparts

APPETITE SUPPRESSANTS	
PRESCRIPTION DRUGS	NATURAL WEIGHT-LOSS ALTERNATIVES
Phentermine, brain peptide inhibitors,* and leptin-related drugs*	Hydroxycitric acid (HCA), 5-HTP, and certain amino acids
FAT-FIGHTERS	
PRESCRIPTION DRUGS	NATURAL WEIGHT-LOSS ALTERNATIVES
Sibutramine (Meridia), beta-3 agonists	Pyruvate, hydroxycitric acid (HCA), carnitine, chromium, guggul, and lipotropics
FAT-BINDERS	
PRESCRIPTION DRUGS	NATURAL WEIGHT-LOSS ALTERNATIVES
Orlistat (Xenical)*	Chitin (an animal fiber), and certain plant fibers
METABOLIC BOOSTERS	
PRESCRIPTION DRUGS	NATURAL WEIGHT-LOSS ALTERNATIVES
Sibutramine (Meridia)	Pyruvate, MCT oil, creatine, carnitine, and ciwujia

*Not approved by the FDA as of spring 1998.

BUYING STANDARDIZED PRODUCTS

Many natural weight-loss supplements are formulated with herbs, or from parts of plants. The better-quality herbal supplements will be "standardized," which means the products have been processed to ensure a uniform level of one or more isolated active ingredients from bottle to bottle.

To standardize a product, the manufacturer extracts key active ingredients from the whole herb, measures them, sometimes concentrates them, and then formulates them in a base with other nutrients, including the whole herb.

Standardization is a good indicator that the product contains the exact amounts to produce the desired results. To check whether a product carries this assurance, you must read the label and look for the ingredients that have been standardized. For example, the label on a bottle of hydroxycitric acid (HCA) might read: "Two capsules provide 2,000 mg standardized garcinia cambogia extract [the herb that contains HCA] supplying 1,000 mg of hydroxycitric acid." Or the label might give a percentage: "Two capsules provide 150 mg of St. John's wort standardized to 0.3% hypericin [the active component in St. John's wort]."

Additionally, you'll need to familiarize yourself with the names of the various active ingredients that are extracted. This book will help you do that.

Standardized products tend to be more expensive than whole or bulk herbs. Still, it's best to buy standardized products so that you know what you're getting.

PART I

NATURAL FAT-FIGHTERS

PYRUVATE: THE BREAKTHROUGH DISCOVERY
THAT REVS UP YOUR FAT-BURNING ENGINE

Suppose there were a safe, natural pill you could pop, and before long, you started losing pounds? Wouldn't you want such a pill in your medicine chest?

Good news: There is such a pill, and you can get it at the health food store. It's pyruvate (pie-RU-vate), a normal constituent of human metabolism. It is also found in many foods in minute amounts, and is truly one of the most fascinating anti-fat supplements around. What's more, pyruvate is one of the most clinically researched and documented weight-loss products on the market.

Since the 1970s, pyruvate has been tested and researched at some of the leading medical centers throughout the world, and has been shown in initial clinical studies to accelerate fat-loss, boost endurance, and work in the body as a disease-fighting antioxidant. It has been available commercially as a supplement only since 1997, and comes in capsule, powder, and drink forms. While some pyruvate supplements are the pure stuff, others contain added ingredients, including herbs, fibers, and certain nutrients— probably because manufacturers are trying to set their particular product apart from the competition. You must read the labels and understand what each formulation contains.

WHAT IS PYRUVATE?

Pyruvate is actually a carbohydrate because it is chemically composed of carbon, hydrogen, and oxygen. Made naturally in the body, pyruvate is involved in the energy-producing reactions that go on in your body at the cellular level. During normal metabolism, carbohydrate fuel (glucose) is split into pyruvate, also known as pyruvic acid, inside individual cells. Pyruvate enters the mitochondria, the energy factory of cells, and undergoes a further series of chemical reactions, ultimately releasing carbon dioxide and water, and producing energy in the form of ATP, a molecular fuel that powers our bodies. ATP makes muscles contract, allows our organs to do their jobs, and promotes other cellular energy processes vital to life. Thus pyruvate is a major natural compound that helps produce energy inside cells.

Pyruvate is also found in many of the foods we eat. Among the richest sources are red Delicious apples, golden Delicious apples, bananas, spinach, red wine, and dark beer. On average, we consume about 500 mg of pyruvate daily from food. The FDA has approved pyruvic acid and its derivatives as additives to enhance the flavor of food.

The dietary supplements sold as pyruvate are derived from tartaric acid, a natural by-product of winemaking. Widely distributed in nature and found in fruits such as grapes, tartaric acid is classified as a fruit acid. It is chemically converted into pyruvic acid during the supplement-manufacturing process. Pyruvic acid, however, is chemically unstable, and produces nausea and intestinal problems when taken in large amounts. To stabilize pyruvic acid and avoid these problems, manufacturers bond it to a mineral salt, usually of calcium or sodium. Because of the chemical processing involved in making pyruvate dietary products, the supplements aren't really "all-natural." More correctly, they are synthetic products made from natural sources.

Taken at suggested doses, pyruvate supplements produce no adverse side effects and yield very desirable metabolic effects—outcomes that have been substantiated by animal and human research.

HOW PYRUVATE WORKS

Much animal research into pyruvate preceded the more recent human clinical trials. Pyruvate's potential was first discovered in the 1970s at the University of Pittsburgh, where a research team led by Dr. Ronald T. Stanko, a physician and professor of medicine, observed some very intriguing effects. In the livers of test animals, pyruvate and dihydroxyacetone, or DHA, a pyruvate-like substance, reduced fatty buildup induced experimentally by excessive alcohol intake. What's more, the rats supplemented with pyruvate and DHA lost abdominal fat.

A point of clarification: In many of the pyruvate studies, researchers used a combination of pyruvate and DHA. There are a couple of reasons for this. The form of pyruvate used in experiments was typically sodium pyruvate, one of the first formulations available. To prevent subjects from consuming too much sodium, DHA was used as part of the test dosages. Also, some studies allowed researchers to compare the effectiveness of pyruvate versus DHA in promoting weight loss. They found that pyruvate was a better agent, hands down.

The early findings on pyruvate led to many more studies on the effects of pyruvate and/or DHA on fat loss. More than a decade of animal studies revealed that these substances did the following:

- Decreased body fat levels by as much as 22 percent

- Reduced the conversion of food calories into body fat (pyruvate was more effective at this than DHA)

- Doubled the use of fat for energy

- Increased metabolism by as much as 30 percent

- Increased metabolically active body protein (muscle) by 20 percent.

Most remarkably, the same weight-loss benefits observed in animals have been found in humans. Let's take a closer look.

Pyruvate May Enhance Fat Loss

Can pyruvate really make fat vanish? Two studies say—yes. In a study published in 1992 in the *American Journal of Clinical Nutrition*, thirteen obese women were placed on a 500-calorie-a-day liquid diet for 3 weeks. Half the women supplemented with 19 grams of pyruvate and 12 grams of DHA; the other half (the control group) received a carbohydrate placebo (a look-alike pill). This was a "double-blind" study, meaning that neither the subjects nor the researchers knew who was receiving the supplement or the placebo.

After three weeks, the pyruvate/DHA-supplemented women lost more weight (14.3 pounds) and body fat (9.5 pounds), compared with their nonsupplemented counterparts, who lost 12.3 pounds of weight and 7.7 pounds of fat. Specifically, that's a 16 percent greater weight loss and a 23 percent better fat loss than those taking the placebo experienced. Another way to put it: The pyruvate combo resulted in a loss of 0.6 extra pound of fat a week.

A second double-blind study, conducted with pyruvate alone, produced an even more impressive fat loss. Fourteen obese women dieted for 3 weeks, consuming a 1,000-calorie-a-day liquid diet. Some of the women supplemented with 36 grams of pyruvate, while the rest took a carbohydrate placebo. The pyruvate-supplemented women lost 37 percent more weight than the controls (13 pounds versus 9.5 pounds). Even better: Pyruvate stimulated a fat loss of 48 percent—the equivalent of almost an extra full pound of pure pudge a week.

Pyruvate Helps Keep Fat Off

If you've ever dieted successfully, you know that maintaining your weight loss is like roller-skating uphill. Astonishingly, pyruvate may help you keep from regaining the weight you worked so hard to lose. In a 1996 study, researchers at the Clinical Research Center at the University of Pittsburgh placed a group of seventeen obese women on a very low-calorie diet (310 calories a day) for 3 weeks. The women, aged 22 to 60, weighed between 160 pounds and 307 pounds. By the end of the diet, they had shed an average of 17.6 pounds of body weight and 11 pounds of body fat.

After the period of dieting, the subjects were placed in two groups. During a second 3-week experimental period, the first group consumed a diet of roughly 2,500 to 2,700 calories a day, including a carbohydrate source of calories. So did the second group—but with a difference: They received a supplement of pyruvate (15 grams) and DHA (75 grams) instead of the carbohydrate.

Here's what happened: All the women regained weight, including body fat. However, the pyruvate/DHA-supplemented women gained 36 percent less weight (4 pounds versus 6.4 pounds) and 55 percent less body fat (1.8 pounds versus 4 pounds).

Of course, this is only one study, but promising nonetheless to millions of people who struggle to keep pounds off permanently.

Pyruvate Changes Your Shape for the Better

Perhaps the most exciting study on pyruvate was conducted in 1997 by a team of researchers from Beth Israel Medical Center in New York City, Yale University School of Medicine, and an independent nutrition research firm. The study enlisted fifty-three people who were toting around 10 to 15 pounds of extra fat—often the hardest flab to budge. They followed a liberal 2,000-calorie diet; performed moderate exercise for 30 minutes a day, 5 days a week; and supplemented with 6 grams of pyruvate a day. There was also a control group, as well as a group who took a placebo.

There are many pyruvate products available; the product used in this study was Pyruvate+, manufactured by New Vision International. While pyruvate is the primary component of the formulation (1,200 mg of pyruvate from sodium and calcium pyruvate), this particular supplement contains other ingredients as well: 10 mg zinc, 3 mg B_6, 100 mcg chromium, 60 mg cornsilk, 20 mg uva ursi, 10 mg cranberry powder, and 10 mg DHA. Cornsilk, uva ursi, and cranberry powder are herbs with a mild diuretic effect. (For more information on these and other diet herbs, see chapter 13.)

The results of this study were spectacular: In six weeks the pyruvate-supplemented people lost 4.8 pounds of pure body fat, a weekly fat loss of 0.8 pound. By contrast, the control group gained 0.1 pound of body fat; the placebo group lost 0.2 pound, on average.

Further, the 4.8 pounds of fat loss is very significant when you consider that the participants were eating 2,000 calories a day and not cutting calories by 500 or 1,000 a day, as in other pyruvate studies or restrictive diets.

Better yet, the pyruvate group gained 3.4 pounds of lean muscle (without engaging in heavy-duty weight training). The control group had a small gain of lean muscle—0.4 pound—and the placebo group lost 0.3 pound of muscle. So basically, the pyruvate supplementers shed unsightly fat and replaced it with curvier, body-firming muscle.

But these were not the only benefits observed with pyruvate supplementation. Those taking the pyruvate product experienced an 18 percent increase in energy levels, compared with increases of 1.8 and 4.5 percent in the control and placebo groups. Also, the pyruvate supplementers' metabolism rose by 2.2 percent.

But how, exactly, does pyruvate work its body-changing, fat-fighting magic? In an excellent guidebook titled *Pyruvate: A Scientific Review and Practical Guide*, James B. Roufs, Ph.D., a leading pyruvate researcher, outlines several possible ways, all based on scientific data and observations.

First, pyruvate may rev up your metabolic rate—the speed at which your body breaks down stored fat and carbohydrate for energy—as the study cited above shows. The faster your metabolic rate, the more efficiently your body burns fat. Even so, it remains a mystery as to why pyruvate may increase metabolism. It may be because pyruvate increases thyroxine, a thyroid hormone. Thyroid hormones are chemical regulators of metabolism; thus, increasing their secretion may boost metabolism.

Second, if pyruvate increases muscle tissue—another effect seen in animal studies and at least one human study—this could account for a higher metabolic rate. Muscle is your body's most metabolically active tissue. For every new pound of muscle you put on, you use about 50 to 100 calories more a day. You can eat more and not gain weight because you burn more, even while sleeping. Poor muscle development, on the other hand, makes it easy for your body to store fat.

A third theory has to do with pyruvate's ability to stimulate fat-burning—an effect observed in both animal and human studies. In normal energy release, the body draws first on carbohydrates for energy, then protein, and finally fat. Remarkably, pyruvate appears to reverse that order, causing your body to burn fat first for its energy needs. Why the reversal? What happens, theoretically, is this: Pyruvate may reduce insulin levels in the blood. Insulin is a busy hormone. Among its duties is promoting fat storage. But if insulin levels are low, less fat is stored in fat cells—which could partially explain pyruvate's effect on fat-burning. More research is needed to confirm these effects.

One final theory involves "feed efficiency," a term that describes how efficiently calories are turned into stored body fat. A high feed efficiency means more calories are stored as fat; a low feed efficiency means fewer calories are deposited. Somehow, pyruvate seems to decrease feed efficiency and prevent excess fat storage; at least, this is what has been observed in animal studies. How pyruvate works this miracle is unclear, but it may enhance calorie-burning mechanisms in the body. It's too early to tell, based on the limited research into pyruvate and feed efficiency, but potentially you could turn yourself into a calorie-burning machine by supplementing with pyruvate.

OTHER REMARKABLE HEALTH BENEFITS

Pyruvate Boosts Energy

Pyruvate can accelerate the body's use of glycogen (stored carbohydrate) by working muscles. It maneuvers more glucose, from the breakdown of glycogen, into cells, where it can be burned for energy. Studies have found that pyruvate increases endurance by up to 20 percent and significantly reduces muscle fatigue—which is why the supplement is so popular among athletes and exercisers.

To date, a couple of studies have looked into the endurance-building benefits of pyruvate. One experiment found that supplementation with very high doses (100 grams) of pyruvate/DHA daily for a week boosted arm endurance by 20 percent. A second study (this one evaluated leg endurance) produced similar results. In fact, supplementation boosted endurance levels more effectively than a diet in which 70 percent of the calories were derived from carbohydrates, the body's preferred fuel source. The broad implication of these findings is that you presumably could do more each day—without pooping out—by supplementing with pyruvate.

Quite possibly, adding pyruvate to your supplement program can help you work out longer and harder. Which, in turn, can help you lose fat—in two key ways. First, exercise burns calories, creating a caloric deficit leading to fat loss as long as you watch what you eat. Second, harder workouts—particularly through strength-developing exercise—help you build muscle. And as noted earlier, the more body-firming muscle you have, the higher your metabolism. A fine-tuned metabolism is one of your best defenses against unwanted fat gain.

Pyruvate Works as an Antioxidant

Antioxidants are vitamins, minerals, enzymes, and other natural chemicals that protect cells from the onslaught of "free radicals." Chemically, a free radical is a molecule that is missing a part of itself—one of its orbiting electrons. To regain stability, the free radical seizes an electron from another molecule or ditches its unpaired one. In the process, the free radical wreaks molecular havoc by boring through cell walls and making it easy for bacteria, viruses, and other disease-causing agents to slip in and do often-irreparable harm.

Antioxidants to the rescue. These heroes simply donate an electron to a free radical but without changing into radicals themselves. This action "neutralizes," or stops, the dangerous multiplication of still more free radicals—a process that if left unchecked could be deadly. Life-shortening diseases such as heart disease, cancer, arthritis, and Alzheimer's disease have all been linked to free-radical damage.

Many factors give rise to these biological terrorists, including normal metabolism, stress, exercise, sunlight, and exposure to environmental toxins such as cigarette smoke, exhaust fumes, and other pollutants. There are different types of free radicals in the body, and some even do good deeds. For instance, cells in our immune system deliberately make free radicals to kill off foreign invaders such as bacteria and viruses.

Normally, free radicals don't cause much of a problem. But when free radicals—even the "good" kind—start outnumbering antioxidants, there's trouble—a condition scientists call "oxidative stress," which leads to disease.

Because there are different types of free radicals, certain antioxidants are uniquely effective against specific radicals—which is why it's a good idea to take a variety of antioxidants, such as beta carotene, vitamin C, vitamin E, selenium, and others.

Pyruvate is particularly effective at neutralizing the hydroxyl radical, a form of hydrogen peroxide. Once generated, this devilish free radical attacks whatever is next to it, setting off a dangerous chain reaction that creates many more free radicals. In a study at the University of Minnesota's School of Medicine, researchers found that pyruvate virtually healed the tissue damage that occurred after rats were given huge doses of hydrogen peroxide. One of the reasons pyruvate is so effective against the hydroxyl radical is that pyruvate, like the radical itself, can easily move in and out of cells. In fact, no other antioxidant can move so freely as pyruvate. Thus, pyruvate is constantly on the trail of this cellular renegade.

Additionally, in an animal study at Cornell University Medical College, researchers were surprised to learn that cells can actually export pyruvate as kind of a protective moat around themselves. Thus, supplementing with pyruvate can be a powerful bodyguard against the multiplication of harmful free radicals.

You may have heard or read that pyruvate is a more effective antioxidant than vitamin E. One animal study did find this to be true; it showed that pyruvate did a better job than vitamin E of inhibiting hydrogen peroxide. But a qualification is in order. Remember, certain antioxidants are effective against specific free radicals. It just so happens that the hydroxyl radical's nemesis is pyruvate. Vitamin E's strength as an antioxidant lies in its ability to defend cell membranes against free-radical attack. The message here is that it is a healthy practice to consume a variety of antioxidants, from both food and supplements.

The studies looking into pyruvate's benefit as an antioxidant have been conducted on animals only, so we don't know what it might do in humans. But if pyruvate can truly fend off the damage done by free radicals, we may have a potentially powerful bodyguard against disease and aging in this supplement.

Pyruvate May Be Heart-Healthy

Every 32 seconds, someone in the United States dies of heart disease. It is the leading killer of both men and women, claiming approximately a million lives each year. Heart disease is also the leading cause of death worldwide. While its toll on human life is staggering, so is its economic impact on society. Currently, heart and blood vessel diseases cost a whopping $164.3 billion a year to treat.

If you're concerned about beating our nation's number-one killer—and who isn't?—you'll be excited about the power and promise of pyruvate.

Pyruvate appears to protect the heart—in at least three possible ways. One is that supplementation may reduce levels of LDL cholesterol (the artery-clogging variety) in the body. In a study of forty middle-aged, obese subjects who followed a high-fat, high-cholesterol diet (similar to what the average American eats) for 6 weeks, the pyruvate-supplemented group reduced their LDL cholesterol by 4 percent, whereas no such change occurred in the placebo-supplemented control group. Of course, this is just a single study—more evidence is needed to confirm pyruvate's possible cholesterol-lowering effect—but a promising study nonetheless.

In addition to LDL cholesterol, another culprit in heart disease is ischemia, a lack of oxygen to the heart that injures heart tissue and can lead to a heart attack. If tissue is labeled "ischemic," this means it lacks a blood supply.

In one study, researchers gave pyruvate to rats whose hearts had been damaged by ischemia. What they found was intriguing: Pyruvate significantly improved the hearts' recovery after supplementation, compared with nonpyruvate-treated hearts. There are two possible explanations for this heart-protective effect. First, the researchers found that pyruvate reduced the formation of superoxide free radicals—a type of free radical that is particularly harmful to the mitochondria in heart cells. Second, pyruvate nearly halted the release of purines from the heart muscle in the treated hearts. Purines are naturally occurring substances in the body. Their release is a signal that the heart muscle has been damaged. There is some anecdotal (unscientific) evidence that pyruvate may heal ischemic heart tissue in humans, but scientific studies are needed to verify this.

In another animal study, pyruvate was shown to improve cardiac function by increasing the amount of blood pumped by the heart, strengthening its ability to contract, and building up the amount of oxygen in the veins.

Of course, much more research into pyruvate's effect on the heart is needed to further document its preliminary promise.

Pryvate May Fight Tumors

The same researchers at the University of Pittsburgh who conducted the pioneering research on pyruvate have also looked into its effect on tumor growth in animals. They implanted rats with breast cancer cells and administered supplemental pyruvate. Pyruvate reduced tumor weight by 40 percent and metastasis (spreading of the tumor) by 42 percent. The tumors also shrank in size. The reasons for these effects are unknown, although the explanation could ultimately lie in pyruvate's ability to fend off free radicals. But more studies are needed to shed light on pyruvate's possible role in treating cancer.

HOW TO USE PYRUVATE

Without a doubt, pyruvate is an exciting supplement. The question is: How much should you take?

The fat-fighting doses of pyruvate used in most of the experimental studies are quite high (28 to 100 grams a day). Using therapeutic megadoses of an experimental substance is customary in scientific research, to detect toxicity and side effects. Even at the very high doses used in studies, few untoward or toxic effects were observed as a result of pyruvate supplementation. In fact, the only side effects experienced were diarrhea and gas, in 10 to 35 percent of the people taking pyruvate.

To determine an appropriate dose, researchers have extrapolated dosages from animal studies to humans, using calculations based on body weight. They have determined that the optimal dose for weight loss and endurance exercise is between 4 and 6 grams a day. The 6-grams-per-day dosage proved to be effective in the 6-week study in which participants lost body fat and gained lean muscle. Studies using lower doses are continuing.

For best results, these amounts should be taken in divided doses every 4 to 6 hours, preferably with meals. Taking pyruvate throughout the day helps maintain higher levels in your body for more efficient action.

Researchers also recommend matching your dosage to your weight. For example, if you weigh between 120 and 165 pounds, an optimal dose would be 4 to 5 grams daily; if you weigh more than 165 pounds, supplement with 5 to 6 grams daily. Current, ongoing studies suggest that you may want to begin with the upper-limit gram dosage until you reach your fat-loss goal, then taper down to a maintenance dose of 2 grams daily for long-term weight management.

Keep in mind, though, that pyruvate has been on the market for only a few years—so we don't know whether it produces any long-term effects. Some health practitioners recommend that you "cycle" your supplementation; that is, take pyruvate for 2 or 3 months while you're dieting, stop taking it for a month, then resume for another 2 or 3 months, and so forth.

Although some people may feel the effects of pyruvate right away, you should give it time to work—in the opinion of researchers, 2 to 3 weeks—before you evaluate its effectiveness in your personal situation. The first time I supplemented with pyruvate, I dropped a few pounds within days. Then—nothing for 2 weeks. By the third week, I had another dramatic loss, for a grand total of 8 pounds in 3 weeks. Also, drinking ample water throughout the day (eight to ten large glasses) seems to help pyruvate work better.

You may feel less hungry when supplementing with pyruvate. This has been my experience, and there are many anecdotal reports of pyruvate's appetite-suppressing effect.

A footnote: Some researchers feel that pyruvate seems to work better the older you are, since the body's supply of pyruvate naturally declines as you age.

PYRUVATE AND DIET

While supplementing with pyruvate, you needn't go on an overly stringent diet. However, if you eat anything you want without regard to calories or fat intake or without exercising, you will only get fatter. Your best bet is to follow a moderate, well-balanced but low-fat diet and exercise plan that decreases your calories by no more than 500 a day, either by exercise, a slight reduction in food, or a combination of the two. Suppose you require an intake of 2,200 calories a day to maintain your weight. To lose fat, you'll need to cut 500 calories daily, for a caloric intake of 1,700 calories a day.

Some researchers feel that pyruvate should be taken with a carbohydrate food, because carbohydrates help pyruvate get into your system more effectively.

Supplementing with pyruvate can potentially enhance your fat-loss efforts and energy systems for more satisfying results. Refer to appendix A for information on planning an appropriate diet.

SAFETY CONSIDERATIONS

Pyruvate is very safe, because it is a natural component of your body's metabolism. Remember, your body makes pyruvate—more specifically, pyruvic acid—on an ongoing basis. Pyruvate causes no harmful side effects when taken in the recommended doses. Nor is it a central nervous stimulant like caffeine, even though it appears to reduce fatigue. Therefore, you'll experience none of the typical side effects associated with stimulants, such as a racing heartbeat, the jitters, or nervousness. Pyruvate is so safe that you don't need a doctor's prescription, although you should always let your physician know if you are taking supplements. And, as with any supplement, if you're diabetic or pregnant or have any medical condition, consult your physician before taking pyruvate.

Currently, pyruvate is available as sodium pyruvate, calcium pyruvate, or a combination of the two. If you take 15 grams of sodium pyruvate, you're adding 3,000 mg of sodium to your diet. The recommended intake of sodium is between 500 mg and 2,400 mg per day, or no more than 1¼ teaspoons of table salt. Therefore, you'd be exceeding the healthy limits for sodium intake. Long-term use of sodium or calcium pyruvate could lead to mineral imbalances.

Fortunately, other forms of pyruvate are in the works. One would combine pyruvate with the amino acid glycine to make pyruvylglycine. This formulation would eliminate the risk of excess sodium intake and possible mineral imbalance. And before long, we may see a supplement that pairs pyruvate with another energizing nutrient, creatine. Such a combo would be of great benefit to athletes and exercisers who want to extend their endurance and increase their training intensities. (For more information on creatine, see chapter 9.)

You can purchase pyruvate in health food stores and pharmacies, or order it from any reputable mail-order supplement company. It is best to buy a product bearing a "MedPro" label. This indicates that the supplement contains a higher amount of pyruvate and is purer. In appendix C, you'll find information on the cost of various pyruvate supplements.

Rating: ★★★★★

REAL-LIFE RESULTS

Deb B., a registered nurse and mother of three, complained of excess fat around her middle after having a hysterectomy. She couldn't seem to shed the weight, no matter what she did. Deb started supplementing with pyruvate, taking two capsules three times a day at meals, according to the supplement manufacturer's directions. She did not exercise, nor did she watch her diet closely.

"Within the first week, I noticed a difference in my waist. It had actually shrunk! Not only could I see this in the mirror, I could feel it every time I got dressed. My clothes were much looser around the waist."

CARNITINE: THE INTERNAL FAT-BURNER
FOR SPEEDIER WEIGHT LOSS

If you want to live the slender life, give your body everything it needs to burn fat efficiently. One way to do that may be through supplementation with a protein-like nutrient called carnitine. Start taking carnitine, and you may find that it's just the supplement you need for more efficient weight loss.

WHAT IS CARNITINE?

In 1905, Russian scientists discovered carnitine in meat. Its name is derived from the word "carnivore," meaning a meat-eating animal. Once thought to be a vitamin and originally named vitamin B_T, carnitine is today considered to be more an amino acid than a vitamin.

Carnitine is the only substance of its kind that can shovel fat into the cells' mitochondria (cellular furnaces) to be burned for energy. It also cleanses the mitochondria by removing waste products. Thus, carnitine is absolutely vital to metabolism. And it has other strong suits. It provides the energy to power the movement of sperm, promotes weight gain in newborns, and helps construct muscle and organ tissues.

A water-soluble nutrient, carnitine is produced in the liver and kidneys from lysine and methionine, two amino acids, through a series of interactions with vitamin C, vitamin B_3, and vitamin B_6. Because your body can make its own carnitine, the nutrient is considered to be nonessential. There is no recommended daily allowance (RDA) for carnitine. In the body, carnitine is concentrated in the skeletal muscle, adrenal glands, and heart muscle—all tissues that rely on fat as their major sources of biological fuel. Although it is found in every cell of our bodies, about 95 percent of the body's carnitine is stored in the muscles. Smaller amounts are distributed in the blood, liver, kidneys, and brain.

If you are obese (weighing more than 20 percent of your normal weight), concentrations of carnitine may be quite high in your liver, according to recent research. This discovery tells us something quite amazing about the human body's ability to adapt. Among the many problems associated with severe obesity is a fatty liver—the liver becomes enlarged due to a buildup of fat within its cells. The liver in its biological wisdom apparently begins producing more carnitine to clear out the excess fat and normalize itself. The liver can do only so much, however. Losing weight will help remove fatty deposits from the liver.

In foods, carnitine is found in red meat (particularly lamb and beef) and other animal products—foods that are typically high in fat. Scientists believe it exists there for a good purpose—to help the body better break down the fat in meat.

Eating red meat supplies a good deal of carnitine. If you chow down on a juicy 8-ounce steak for dinner, for example, you'll get roughly 120 mg of carnitine. Eating the same amount of chicken will give you about 15 mg of carnitine. There is also some carnitine in nuts, avocados, breast milk, dairy products, and grains. On average, we consume between 50 mg and 300 mg of this nutrient a day through food alone. Carnitine is quite vulnerable to heat and is easily destroyed by cooking.

A carnitine deficiency is rare but life-threatening, causing progressive weakness of the heart and other muscles. "Primary carnitine deficiency" is caused by the inability of the body to manufacture the nutrient; "secondary carnitine deficiency" is due to insufficient carnitine in the diet. Some medical experts feel that certain types of obesity are related to a genetic inability to produce enough carnitine. Those at risk of a carnitine deficiency include vegetarians who eat no meat, people with severe burns or injuries, kidney disease patients on dialysis, and premature babies.

Carnitine is available both as a natural supplement from health food stores and as the prescription drug Carnitor® (levocarnitine), manufactured by Sigma-Tau Pharmaceuticals, Italy's largest drug company (with a U.S. subsidiary located in Maryland). Carnitor® is the only version of levocarnitine approved by the FDA to treat carnitine deficiency. According to a 1997 article in *Chemical Market Reporter*, there is growing worldwide demand for carnitine, a result of advancing knowledge of the nutrient's potential therapeutic benefits in health and medicine.

HOW CARNITINE WORKS

Carnitine May Help You Burn More Fat

You have about 20 to 30 billion fat cells in your body. Some of this fat is a structural constituent of the brain, nerve tissue, bone marrow, heart, cell membranes, and other tissues and organs. The rest forms "storage fat"—the extra pounds nobody wants but almost everyone has. Some storage fat pads your organs for protection. But most is found just underneath your skin. When you put on fat pounds, storage fat cells become stuffed with fat and enlarge as a result. If you gain 50 pounds or more, fat cells start to multiply, and you've got them for life. Dieting doesn't obliterate fat cells, it only shrinks them. Fat cells fight to keep their size, even when you go on a diet. Some exciting preliminary research conducted with animals shows that carnitine can stop the growth of fat cells and shrink their diameter. If the same response is duplicated in human fat cells, carnitine could turn out to a fat-fighting knight in shining armor!

But carnitine has already demonstrated its fat-fighting power, particularly when combined with chromium picolinate. This dynamic duo appears to boost fat loss—potentially up to 2 or more pounds a week. In one study, thirty obese women and ten obese men were placed on diets (1,200 calories a day for women and 1,600 calories a day for men) while receiving either daily supplements of l-carnitine (200 mg) and chromium picolinate (200 mcg) or a placebo for eight weeks.

The results were remarkable: On average, the supplemented group lost 15 pounds, compared with no weight loss in the placebo group. What's more, the supplemented group lost an average of 3.5 percent body fat, while the other group gained 0.6 percent body fat.

Carnitine May Curb Hunger

Carnitine may moonlight as an appetite suppressant. Quite possibly, you'll be better able to tolerate a low-calorie diet if you're supplementing with carnitine, some medical experts believe. What happens, theoretically, is this: By making fatty acids more available for energy, carnitine reduces hunger pangs and fatigue that result from less efficient fat-burning. Experiments are needed to verify this benefit, however.

Carnitine Energizes You for Exercise

Carnitine has been found to boost exercise performance by making more fat available to working muscles. This is certainly good news if you're active and want to combust fat faster. According to several scientific studies, supplementation causes more fatty acids to enter cells to be used as energy. The more fat available for energy, the better your stamina and performance.

Researchers in Romania gave carnitine to 110 top athletes (rowers, kayakers, swimmers, weight lifters, and long-distance runners) and found the supplementation caused more fatty acids to enter cells to be used as energy. With a larger amount of fat available for energy, performance conceivably can be improved. Based on their findings, the researchers recommended carnitine supplementation as an ergogenic (performance-enhancing) aid, especially for endurance and strength sports.

Another Romanian study looked into the effects of carnitine supplementation on competitive junior cyclists. Seven top cyclists were given 2 grams of carnitine daily 10 days prior to competition, along with extra protein (1 gram per kg of body weight) for 6 weeks; seven other cyclists received a placebo. Favorable changes were observed in the supplemented group: Strength went up, lean muscle increased, and body fat was scaled back. What's more, the supplemented group performed better than the placebo group in the international competition that took place at the end of the experiment. For competitive athletes, the researchers recommend increasing protein intake 6 weeks before competition and supplementing with 2 grams of carnitine daily 10 to 14 days before competing, including the day of competition. Carnitine, they believe, improves the "biological potential" of the body.

But carnitine may not always do the trick. A group of researchers in Switzerland gave 2 grams of l-carnitine, or a placebo, to seven male marathoners 2 hours prior to their marathon run and again after 20 kilometers into the run. Supplementation with carnitine did not improve the runners' performance.

A study of rugby players tested carnitine alone and in combination with caffeine. The players were fed 11 mg of caffeine per pound of body weight and 15 grams of carnitine, then tested on a series of cycling bouts to see how long they could last before tiring out. Both carnitine by itself and with caffeine proved useful. The players were able to exercise longer before fatigue set in. Another interesting finding: The athletes burned more fat during exercise when supplementing with carnitine and with the carnitine/caffeine duo. Like carnitine, caffeine is believed to mobilize fatty acids during exercise. But supplementing with caffeine in the amounts used in this experiment (up to 22 cups of coffee) is not very practical. Excessive consumption of caffeine has harmful side effects, such as dehydration, insomnia, headaches, nervousness, and possibly irregular heartbeats. So forget the coffee and stick with carnitine.

Some scientists believe that carnitine enhances exercise performance in other ways. Evidence is surfacing that carnitine increases VO_2 max (the ability of your body to take in, transport, and use oxygen) and reduces the buildup of waste products like lactic acid in the muscles, thereby extending performance and stamina.

The bottom line: If carnitine supplementation improves aerobic performance—which a growing number of studies say it does—then you could exercise aerobically with greater intensity and thus potentially incinerate more fat.

OTHER REMARKABLE HEALTH BENEFITS

Carnitine Improves Heart Health

Studies on carnitine's role in cardiovascular health began as early as 1937. In fact, a whole book could be devoted to carnitine's beneficial effect on the heart. This hard-working organ prefers to burn fat for fuel. Carnitine acts like a fuel injection system, supplying heart mitochondria with fat for fuel. But trouble starts when the heart muscle is damaged in some way, such as a lack of oxygen, inflammation, obstruction of blood flow, or irregular heartbeats—and its carnitine supply is depleted.

In scores of cases, heart patients have responded well to supplemental carnitine, with subsequent relief of their symptoms. Carnitine can control heart-rhythm irregularities, reduce angina attacks, lower triglycerides (fatty compounds that endanger heart health), decrease harmful LDL cholesterol, and increase helpful HDL cholesterol. Plus, carnitine increases the effectiveness of antioxidants known to help the heart. Quite possibly, carnitine may be one of the most effective heart-health breakthroughs to date, with the power to restore normal heart function.

Carnitine May Boost Immunity to Disease

At least one study shows that carnitine appears to increase the activity of lymphocytes, infection-fighting white blood cells, and to prevent suppression of the immune system. With stronger immunity, you can better protect yourself against illness.

Carnitine May Lessen the Symptoms of Alzheimer's Disease

Carnitine promotes the uptake of the B-vitamin choline by cells and its subsequent formation into acetylcholine, a substance that transmits nerve impulses. Because patients with Alzheimer's disease are deficient in acetylcholine, scientists have speculated that carnitine supplementation may prove of some benefit.

A team of researchers in Italy studied 130 Alzheimer's patients, randomly assigning them to receive 2 grams of carnitine daily or a placebo for a year. By the end of the study, all the patients had deteriorated in mental function. But those who supplemented with carnitine had less deterioration, particularly in memory, attention span, and verbal abilities. This study and others in Europe sparked worldwide interest in carnitine supplementation for treating Alzheimer's disease. Research has intensified and is now ongoing.

HOW TO USE CARNITINE

To encourage fat loss, supplement your diet with 1,000 mg to 1,200 mg of carnitine a day or you may take it in divided doses— 500 mg or 600 mg in the morning and again at night. Some people get good results by taking the entire daily dose 30 to 45 minutes prior to exercise. Use carnitine in conjunction with a low-fat, high-protein, moderate-carbohydrate diet (see "Real Life Results," page 37). This nutrient is available in capsules and in liquid form. It is also an ingredient in other natural weight-loss supplements.

SAFETY CONSIDERATIONS

Supplemental carnitine produces no negative side effects, even in high doses. In fact, the only side effect reported with carnitine supplementation has been a mild state of euphoria.

A word of caution: Like many amino acids, carnitine comes in two forms, called the d- and l-series. L-carnitine is safe because it is the same natural form found in animal or plant tissue. Plus, only the l-form is biologically active. By contrast, the d-form is inactive and unnatural. Some supplement preparations contain a mixture of l-carnitine and d-carnitine. They are cheaper to mass-produce, but are much less effective and not without side effects. A case in point: In one study, patients with cardiac disease who supplemented with l-carnitine were able to exercise longer and with greater aerobic strength than those taking the dl-form. In fact, dl-carnitine decreased exercise performance.

D-carnitine can cause muscle weakness and excretion of myoglobin, the oxygen-transporting protein the blood. So be sure to use products that contain l-carnitine only. Another safe form is acetyl l-carnitine.

Doses over and above those that are recommended may cause gastrointestinal discomfort. Also, people with kidney disease or other illnesses should not supplement with carnitine before conferring with a physician.

Rating: ★★★

REAL-LIFE RESULTS: A SPORTS NUTRITIONIST LOOKS AT L-CARNITINE

Stripping a person's body fat down to superlean proportions—that's part of Todd Swinney's job as a sports nutritionist. And to do it successfully, one of the nutritional tools he uses is l-carnitine.

"I recommend l-carnitine for two reasons. First, it helps shuttle fats into the cells' mitochondria to be burned as fuel. And second, carnitine assists muscles in taking up nutrients called branched-chain amino acids, or BCAAs. These are the amino acids leucine, valine, and isoleucine. An increase of BCAAs in the muscle helps firm the body and possibly enhances muscle growth," explains Todd, who is also a certified professional fitness trainer, certified sports nutritionist, and author of many articles for major fitness magazines.

"Although the body manufactures some carnitine on its own, less is produced when you restrict calories to lose body fat. So supplementation is an excellent way to increase carnitine levels to stoke fat-burning fires."

Todd points out that many natural weight-loss products contain l-carnitine, but usually not in quantities high enough to make a difference in body-fat reduction. "According to research, the minimum dosage required to preserve lean muscle while accelerating fat loss is 1,000 to 1,200 mg daily, divided into two doses. Further research has shown the most effective dose, particularly for athletes, may be 2 to 4 grams in three to six daily doses taken at 3-to-6-hour intervals."

Todd works with a variety of clients, from people hoping to shed some fat pounds for the swimsuit season to competitive bodybuilders who must reduce their body fat to under 5 percent for contests. With competitive bodybuilders, he recommends that they take 1,200 mg of l-carnitine on an empty stomach, 30 to 45 minutes before they perform morning aerobics. During this time, carbohydrate availability is typically low, and so the body starts mobilizing fats for energy. Carnitine helps make even more fat available. The net effect is a greater proportion of fat burned. He advises taking another 1,200 mg 30 to 45 minutes before weight-training, and the same dose again before an evening aerobics session.

But what if you're not a bodybuilder?

"Often, I recommend the same dosages for nonathletes, as long as they exercise regularly. But if a lower dose such as 1,000 mg or 1,200 mg is working, I'll stick with that. As bodybuilders do, it's best to take carnitine in divided doses 30 to 45 minutes prior to exercise."

Diet is critical, too. Todd has found that the best ratio of nutrients for fat-burning is 40 to 45 percent of daily calories from low-fat protein, 50 percent from carbohydrates, and 5 to 10 percent from fat. He also recommends combining carnitine with other lipotropic nutrients, including choline and inositol, to keep fats mobile in the bloodstream so they can burned off.

Using carnitine, diet, and other nutritional supplements, Todd has helped bodybuilders, women fitness competitors, and football players achieve superior physique results and consequent success in their respective sports.

THREE

CHROMIUM: THE MIRACLE MINERAL
THAT FIGHTS FAT GAIN

From pills to powders, hundreds of supplements, including many for weight loss, contain a trace mineral called chromium. Some 10 million people buy roughly $150 million worth of chromium each year, making it the hottest-selling mineral in the country after calcium. And no wonder. Chromium has been touted as a fat-burner, appetite suppressant, muscle builder, energy booster, diabetes preventive, an anti-aging nutrient, and more. But does it live up to its reputation?

The evidence for many of these claims is conflicting, making chromium one of the most controversial supplements around. In fact, the Federal Trade Commission (FTC), the government's advertising watchdog, has gone on record that companies selling chromium do not have adequate scientific evidence to back up the many claims being made for it. As a result, Nutrition 21, the manufacturer and license holder of one form of chromium supplement, agreed in 1997 to notify distributors to stop using promotional materials that make unsubstantiated claims about chromium.

Because chromium is a constituent of many natural weight-loss supplements, it is important for you to know as much as possible about this nutrient—what it can and cannot do, and whether it should be a part of your supplement program.

WHAT IS CHROMIUM?

Chromium's assignment in the body is to help turn carbohydrates into glucose (blood sugar), the fuel burned by cells for energy. Chromium also helps regulate and produce the hormone insulin. Manufactured by the pancreas, insulin helps control hunger, regulates fat storage and muscle-building, and assists the body in utilizing cholesterol properly. Chromium makes insulin work more efficiently in the body. Without chromium, insulin simply would not function.

Like calcium, iron, zinc, and other minerals, chromium is absolutely vital to good health. Yet your body requires it in only the tiniest amounts (50 to 200 micrograms daily). Dietary sources include brewer's yeast, nuts, cheeses, whole-grain cereals, meats, raw oysters, mushrooms, apples with skin, wine, and beer. Despite its presence in food, nine out of ten Americans are deficient in chromium—for the following reasons:

- The chromium found in foods is not easily absorbed by the body. In fact, only about 1 to 3 percent is absorbed.

- To get the minimum amount of chromium required (50 micrograms), you would have to eat between 3,000 and 4,000 calories a day, according to the U.S. Department of Agriculture.

- Diets high in sugar and processed foods (like Western diets) rob the body of chromium. In one study, thirty-seven people (nineteen men and eighteen women) were fed healthy diets with optimal levels of protein, carbohydrates, fat, and other nutrients for 12 weeks. Afterward, for 6 weeks, the subjects were put on a high-sugar diet (15 percent of the total calories were from simple sugars). In twenty-seven of the thirty-seven subjects, the high-sugar diet practically flushed chromium out of their bodies. Clearly, too much sugar in the diet can lead to a chromium deficiency, possibly interfering with your body's ability to use glucose properly and to burn fat.

- Strenuous exercise forces chromium from the body. When you exercise, rather large amounts of chromium are moved into circulation. The proof of this is in studies in which scientists have found that urinary chromium losses are the highest on workout days.

- Food processing and preparation destroy up to 80 percent of the chromium in whole foods.

- Plants do not need chromium to live, so very little is available in the foods we eat.

Supplementally, there are several forms of chromium. Each varies in bioavailability—how easily it is absorbed and retained by the body—and biological activity—how effectively it helps insulin do its job. Chromium is available in several forms.

- **Chromium picolinate.** The best-known form of chromium, chromium picolinate is a patented compound sold under various brand names. Picolinate, or picolinic acid, is a breakdown product of the amino acid tryptophan. When combined with chromium, picolinic acid enhances its absorption.

Most of the research involving chromium has been done with chromium picolinate. However, little is known about how it actually works. Some studies suggest that picolinic acid may affect the central nervous system (the brain and spinal cord). Compounds structurally similar to picolinic acid have been shown to alter the metabolism of the brain chemicals serotonin, dopamine, and norepinephrine— all factors in appetite control.

- **Niacin-bound chromiums** (chromium nicotinate, chromium polynicotinate, and chromium GTF). Chemically tied to the B-vitamin niacin, niacin-bound chromium is the active ingredient in brewer's yeast, one of the richest and best-absorbed sources of biologically active chromium in nature.

In a study at the University of California at Davis, animals fed chromium nicotinate absorbed and retained 311 percent more chromium than those given chromium picolinate and 672 percent more than those given chromium chloride. Some authorities, however, contend that chromium nicotinate is not as effective as chromium picolinate in moving glucose into muscle cells.

Chromium GTF is a complex of nutrients that combines chromium with the B-vitamin niacin and the amino acids cysteine, glycine, and glutamic acid. It is thought to help control hunger and optimize the metabolism of carbohydrates.

- **Chromium chloride.** Multivitamin and mineral supplements are often formulated with chromium chloride. Reportedly, it is not absorbed well (only 0.5 to 2 percent). Also, chromium chloride has little effect on insulin because it must first be converted into a more biologically active form—a process the body has a limited capacity to accomplish.

HOW CHROMIUM WORKS

Chromium and Fat Loss

Several studies conducted in the late 1980s and early 1990s found that daily supplements of either 200 mcg or 400 mcg of chromium picolinate may improve body composition (ratio of fat to muscle) and promote weight loss in healthy adults. One of the very first studies found that supplementing with 200 mcg of chromium picolinate a day promoted fat loss *without dieting or exercise.*

In another study, a group of young male athletes took chromium picolinate while a control group took a placebo. By the end of 6 weeks, the chromium-supplemented group had lost 22 percent of their body fat, contrasted with only a 6 percent loss in the placebo group.

In a separate study, a team of investigators in San Antonio, Texas, recruited two sets of volunteers, ranging in age from 36 to 55 years. For about 10 weeks, the volunteers swilled two nutritional beverages each day that contained either a placebo or 200 mcg or 400 mcg a day of chromium picolinate. They did not change their diets or exercise activity.

No one in the placebo group experienced any significant changes in body composition. But the volunteers who supplemented with chromium picolinate lost an average of 4.2 pounds and gained an average of 1.4 pounds of lean muscle. Also, the older volunteers fared the best. Those supplementing with 400 mcg lost the most weight. This response isn't so surprising, really—we all tend to be chromium-deficient as we age. Supplementing with chromium somehow bolstered the older volunteers' fat-burning ability.

In a study published in the *Journal of the American College of Sports Medicine* in 1996, forty collegiate swimmers (men and women) supplemented with either 400 mcg of chromium or a placebo during their 6-month competitive season. By the end of the season, body-fat losses and muscle gains were 20 to 40 percent higher among the supplementers than among those in the placebo group. The female swimmers taking chromium lost the most fat and gained the most muscle.

Taken together, this collection of studies is pretty convincing that chromium may give a boost to fat loss. But how? There are five possible explanations, according to research:

1. Chromium may increase the power of insulin to undertake another one of its jobs—producing serotonin, a brain chemical that decreases the appetite. Also, since chromium prevents roller-coaster swings in blood sugar, it may diminish the desire to eat and reduce cravings for sweets.

2. Chromium may stimulate the burning of carbohydrates so that they are converted into energy given off as heat, rather than being turned into body fat. Thus, by supplementing with chromium, you may be able to prevent unwanted fat gain. But to shed existing fat, you still have to watch your diet and exercise regularly.

3. Chromium may help regulate the body's fat-producing processes. If you eat too many carbohydrates, your body overproduces insulin. Insulin triggers the activity of lipoprotein lipase, an enzyme that tells fat cells to store fat. But by making insulin work better, chromium in effect prevents excess fat from forming.

4. Chromium may stimulate the metabolism. Some scientists think chromium may jump-start metabolism in brown fat—the special fat that burns stored white fat.

5. Chromium may stimulate protein (muscle) synthesis. For growth and repair of tissues, including muscle, cells need amino acids. Assisted by chromium, insulin helps amino acids gain access to cells. Once inside, amino acids reassemble themselves to construct new muscle tissue. Thus, chromium may have an indirect effect on muscle growth. And the more muscle you have, the less fat you're likely to gain.

Chromium and Body Composition

Other evidence suggests that chromium definitely stimulates the growth of lean muscle if you lift weights. In one study, ten college men attending a strength-training class twice a week took either chromium supplements (200 mcg a day) or a placebo. After 40 days, the chromium supplementers had gained an average of 4.84 pounds of muscle, without gaining any fat. The placebo group did not fare as well. They gained barely a pound of muscle, on average, and their body fat increased by 1.1 percent.

In a study of thirty-one college football players participating in a strength-training program four times a week for 6 weeks, half the group took 200 mcg a day of chromium, while the other half took a placebo. By the end of the experimental period, the chromium-supplemented players had lost 3.6 percent body fat and gained 5.7 pounds of muscle. The placebo group lost only 1.2 percent fat and gained 4 pounds of lean muscle mass.

However, more recent studies say the chromium picolinate's fat-fighting power may not be all it's cracked up to be. A few examples follow.

At the University of Massachusetts, thirty-six football players were given either a placebo or 200 mcg of chromium picolinate daily for 9 weeks during spring training—a period in which they worked out with weights and engaged in a running program. Before, during, and after supplementation, the researchers assessed the players' diet, urinary chromium losses, girth of various body parts, percentages of body fat and muscle, and strength. Percentages of body fat and muscle were measured by underwater weighing, one of the most precise methods to gauge body composition. The findings: Chromium supplementation did not help build muscle, enhance strength, or burn fat.

Several years ago, the United States Navy looked into whether chromium picolinate could be used to help its personnel shed fat. At the Naval Health Research Center in San Diego, California, investigators enrolled ninety-five healthy, active-duty personnel (seventy-nine men and sixteen women) in a scientific experiment to put the supplement to the test. All the participants exceeded the Navy's body-fat standards of 22 percent for men and 30 percent for women.

For 16 weeks, they took either 400 mcg of chromium picolinate or a placebo daily and participated in a physical conditioning program that included aerobic exercise three times a week for at least 30 minutes each session. By the end of the study, the entire group had lost a small amount of weight and a little body fat. There were no significant losses among the supplementers. The Navy concluded that chromium picolinate didn't work well to encourage fat loss, and decided not to recommend it as a diet aid in its weight-reduction programs.

One of the biggest surprises regarding chromium emerged in a study published in 1997: Chromium nicotinate appeared to have more of an effect on weight loss than chromium picolinate did. At the University of Texas at Austin, researchers wanted to know what effect chromium supplementation had on certain risk factors for heart disease and diabetes, particularly body weight and body composition. In this study, young obese women supplemented with 400 mcg daily of either chromium picolinate or chromium nicotinate, combined with exercise. The women supplementing with chromium picolinate actually gained weight, whereas the other group lost a significant amount of weight.

Obviously, the jury is still out as to whether chromium plays a role in enhancing fat loss and improving body composition. Many authorities do agree on one point, however: If you're chromium-deficient, you may experience some benefit.

Which brings up another question: How do you know whether you're deficient? A lab test may detect chromium levels in your body, and some health-care professionals recommend hair analysis. The most reliable gauge, however, may be your lifestyle. Anyone who routinely eats a high-sugar diet or exercises extensively may be at risk. And, as noted above, chromium levels decline with age.

Deficiency symptoms often mimic those of diabetes: overweight, abnormal thirst, frequent urination, fatigue, increased appetite, decreased immunity, and yeast infections.

OTHER REMARKABLE HEALTH BENEFITS

Chromium and Diabetes

Sometimes normal insulin activity becomes upset, and the cells can't use glucose properly. Either not enough insulin is produced (a condition known as Type I diabetes) or the cells aren't letting in enough glucose for proper nourishment (Type II diabetes). Chromium may be a part of the medical solution.

Decades of research show that chromium supplementation helps lessen and even reverse the symptoms of diabetes, particularly Type II diabetes. The reasons for this are clear: Chromium helps insulin regulate and normalize blood sugar, and also decreases insulin requirements. In addition, it improves the body's ability to transport blood glucose into cells for energy.

Chromium and Cardiovascular Disease

Chromium supplementation has been found to reduce dangerous LDL cholesterol and triglycerides in the body—both risk factors for heart disease. Additionally, chromium raises levels of heart-protecting HDL cholesterol. In studies, chromium picolinate and chromium nicotinate have both been found to lower cholesterol levels. Thus, chromium supplementation may be of nutritional significance in preventing and treating heart disease.

Chromium and Osteoporosis

Osteoporosis is a painful thinning of the bones that can afflict women after menopause. It causes disfigurement, disability, and broken bones. Fortunately, it's preventable—particularly with a healthy, calcium-rich diet and exercise. A couple of studies have found that supplements of either chromium picolinate or chromium chloride have prevented bone loss. Researchers, however, feel that chromium probably works best in concert with other minerals, and not on its own.

HOW TO USE CHROMIUM

Despite the fact that chromium has been in the spotlight for a long time, no one really knows exactly how much chromium we need. Although benefits of chromium supplementation have been reported at levels ranging from 200 to 400 mcg daily, the National Academy of Science suggests 50 mcg to 200 mcg daily as a guideline for healthy adults. Chromium is best taken once or twice a day, with meals, since food aids in the absorption of minerals.

Chromium researchers who support its use as a weight-loss aid say it takes at least 8 weeks of supplementation (200 mcg to 400 mcg daily) before you see results.

The cost of chromium varies widely from store to store. You may pay anywhere from $6 to $9 for a bottle of sixty chromium tablets. It's best to shop around and purchase supplements from better-known manufacturers. Prices of various chromium products are listed in appendix C.

Chromium supplements may contain other ingredients, including l-carnitine, HCA, and herbs. No one really knows for sure whether adding other ingredients makes chromium more effective. Also, some supplements may contain more than the recommended safe limit of 200 mcg. Read the label to know what you're buying.

CHROMIUM AND DIET

Like most natural weight-loss supplements, chromium works best if lifestyle changes are made. If you supplement with chromium for weight control, it is advisable to eat a low-fat, low-sugar, high-fiber diet. Also, the scientific data on chromium supplementation suggest that the supplement may significantly improve fat loss and alter body composition favorably when combined with regular exercise, particularly aerobics and strength-developing exercise.

SAFETY CONSIDERATIONS

Debate swirls around the safety of supplementing with chromium. Thus, there are some yellow cautionary traffic lights regarding chromium supplementation and its effect on health. A study released in 1995 suggested that supplementation may damage chromosomes, the bodies inside the cell nucleus that carry our genes. In the laboratory, researchers injected hefty amounts of chromium picolinate into hamster cells in dishes—about 3,000 times the safe amount you'd see in people supplementing with 200 mcg a day. The chromosomes broke, and such breakage can lead to cancer. Other forms of chromium, chromium nicotinate, and chromium chloride, did not cause this damage.

Defenders of chromium picolinate responded by pointing out that the study was meaningless because such high doses of chromium were used. Moreover, it's not reasonable to extrapolate any meaning from cells in dishes to live human beings. Even the researchers admitted their findings were inconclusive and warrant further investigation.

Another concern involves iron deficiency. If you're at risk of an iron shortage, be cautious about supplementing with chromium. Like two passengers trying to hop in the same taxi, chromium competes with iron at a critical site in the hemoglobin-making process. (Hemoglobin is a protein in red blood cells that carries oxygen around the body.) Thus, iron can't do its job of manufacturing hemoglobin if chromium interferes. This has led to speculation as to whether chromium adversely affects iron status in the body. There's no clear-cut answer, however. One study found that men taking chromium picolinate had less iron in a protein that carries iron into the bone marrow, where it is used to manufacture new blood cells. Another study found that supplementation with chromium picolinate didn't affect iron status at all.

Leading chromium researchers agree that it is very safe when taken at the recommended levels (50 mcg to 200 mcg daily). What's more, chromium has a very low toxicity. But extra-high doses of chromium can build up in the liver and kidneys, and potentially can cause damage. Doses of more than 600 mcg a day may cause heart arrhythmias, nervousness, or liver and kidney damage.

If you have diabetes or lung, liver, or kidney disease, consult with your doctor before supplementing. As with most supplements, it's advisable to avoid chromium supplementation if you are pregnant or breast-feeding.

Rating: ★★★★

LIPOTROPICS: FAT-MOBILIZING NUTRIENTS

Although lipotropics may be the oldest natural weight-loss supplements on the market, they're experiencing a resurgence in popularity, especially as prescription diet pills continue to lose favor with dieters. Technically, "lipotropic" refers to any substance that decreases the rate at which fat is stored in liver cells and accelerates the rate at which fat is dismantled into water, carbon dioxide, and energy during metabolism.

WHAT ARE LIPOTROPICS?

Lipotropic supplements contain nutrients that may help prevent fat from accumulating faster than your body can use it. They do not, however, substitute for proper diet and regular exercise. If you are currently overweight and the only change you make in your lifestyle is to supplement with lipotropics, most likely nothing will happen.

Nor do lipotropic supplements burn fat, contrary to what many supplement manufacturers claim. All lipotropic supplements do is provide a precise combination of nutrients your body needs to metabolize fat at the maximum rate—as long as you are following a low-fat, high-nutrient diet and are exercising regularly.

Many nutrients are classified as lipotropics, including chromium, carnitine, the amino acid methionine, and certain herbs, all explained elsewhere in the book. Others are members of the B-complex family of vitamins. These are covered here.

VITAMIN B₅ (PANTOTHENIC ACID)

The name pantothenic acid comes from the Greek word *pantothen*, which means "everywhere"—an apt derivativation, since this B-complex vitamin is present in every living cell. First recognized as a substance that stimulates growth, pantothenic acid is quite active in metabolism. It is a building block of CoA, a key enzyme that releases energy from foods. Pantothenic acid stimulates the adrenal glands and boosts production of hormones responsible for healthy skin and nerves. It guards the health of the digestive tract. Additionally, pantothenic acid is involved in immunity, wound healing, the formation of hormones, and the regulation of nerve impulses.

At Hong Kong Central Hospital in China, pantothenic acid has been given to overweight-to-obese patients put on a medically supervised low-calorie diet. Noting good results with supplementation, the medical team there has hypothesized that supplementation with pantothenic acid promotes the complete burning, or breakdown, of fatty acids while preventing ketosis. Ketosis is an undesirable condition in which by-products of fat breakdown accumulate in the blood. It disturbs the blood's normal chemistry by making the blood more acidic, and high blood acidity interferes with the normal function of cells. Because pantothenic acid is vital for the proper synthesis of fatty acids, this hypothesis may have some validity. Suffice it to say that more information needs to be uncovered about the exact role pantothenic acid plays in fat-burning.

Foods rich in pantothenic acid include organ meats, brewer's yeast, egg yolks, and whole grains. Cooking and food processing destroy up to 50 percent (sometimes more) of the vitamin.

Pantothenic acid is so widespread in foods, however, that deficiencies are usually not a problem. In addition, the vitamin can be made in the body by intestinal bacteria. Many multivitamin supplements contain pantothenic acid. The recommended daily intake for adults is 4 to 7 mg.

Rating: ★

VITAMIN B₆ (PYRIDOXINE)

Vitamin B_6 is a component of many natural weight-loss supplements—for several reasons. First, vitamin B_6 aids in the conversion of the amino acids tyrosine and phenylalanine into brain neurotransmitters that, among other functions, help suppress the appetite. (See chapter 7 for more information on amino acids.) Second, vitamin B_6 helps maintain the balance of sodium and potassium in cells—a balance necessary to regulate fluids properly. Thus, vitamin B_6 indirectly helps prevent water retention, a condition that can make you look and feel fat. Taking 100 mg of vitamin B_6 one to three times a day is often recommended to reduce fluid buildup. Third, vitamin B_6 helps regulate blood sugar. Swings in blood sugar can lead to food cravings and low energy. Finally, restrictive diets can deplete the body's supply of vitamin B_6, and supplementation is extra insurance against a deficiency. Clearly, this nutrient is a behind-the-scenes player in many issues related to weight management.

Vitamin B_6 influences nearly every system in the body. For example, it assists in metabolizing fats, creating amino acids (the building blocks of protein), turning carbohydrates into glucose, producing neurotransmitters (brain chemicals that relay messages), and manufacturing antibodies to ward off infection.

Also, vitamin B_6 (along with folic acid) is needed to prevent the buildup of homocysteine, a toxic by-product of the amino acid methionine, in the blood. Homocysteine causes the cells lining arterial walls to deteriorate. In response, the arteries start rebuilding by creating new cells and new connective tissue that attract fats such as cholesterol and triglycerides. This reconstructive process can eventually lead to atherosclerosis, a buildup of fatty substances within artery walls.

If you're active, you may be interested in knowing that extra vitamin B_6 can help boost endurance. Research has demonstrated that supplemental B_6 may improve VO_2 max, a measurement of the body's ability to use oxygen.

The best food sources of vitamin B_6 include salmon, Atlantic mackerel, white meat of chicken, halibut, tuna, broccoli, lentils, and brown rice.

If you're simultaneously supplementing with a natural weight-loss product *and* a multivitamin pill that both contain vitamin B_6, make sure you're not getting too much of a good thing. The recommended daily intake for vitamin B_6 is 2 mg for every 100 grams of protein you eat, roughly the amount in a chicken breast. The average multivitamin pill contains 1.7 mg; single supplements of vitamin B_6 may contain as much as 100 mg.

High doses of vitamin B_6 can be dangerous. Years ago, it was reported that women taking more than 2 grams daily for two months or more for PMS symptoms experienced worrisome health problems, including numbness in their feet and loss of sensation in their hands. The problems subsided when the women stopped taking the supplements. The message here: Always read supplement labels, calculate how much of certain nutrients you're taking in, and never megadose.

Rating: ★★

BIOTIN

This B-complex vitamin is required to activate specific enzymes involved in metabolism. Without it, the body can't properly burn fats— which is why you so often find biotin as an ingredient in natural weight-loss products. It also affects the body's ability to metabolize blood properly.

In addition, biotin helps the body utilize protein and is involved in the metabolism of keratin, the hard protein in nails. If your fingernails are brittle, biotin may be just the remedy you need (it heals and hardens the hooves of pigs and horses). Research shows that supplementing with biotin thickens fingernails and keeps their outer layers from peeling off. Biotin's benefit to nails is the reason you find the vitamin in beauty supplements sold at the cosmetics counter.

Although required in tiny amounts (150 to 300 mcg daily), biotin can be in short supply—for two reasons. First, the best sources of biotin in food are egg yolks and liver, two foods we tend to cut out because of their high concentration of cholesterol.

Second, research verifies that active people often have lower levels of biotin than those who are sedentary. One theory is related to exercise. Exercising causes the waste product lactic acid to accumulate in working muscles. Biotin helps break down lactic acid. The more lactic acid that builds up in muscles, the more biotin that's needed to break it down. If you're a regular exerciser, supplementing with biotin—either through a multivitamin formula or a lipotropic supplement—offers an extra measure of protection against a possible shortfall.

Even so, deficiencies are rare, and one reason is that biotin can be manufactured by bacteria in the intestines. It is also distributed in small amounts in animal and plant foods such as milk, liver, egg yolks, whole grains, and soy flour. Years ago, it was believed that people who ate little or no animal products would be at risk for deficiencies. But a fascinating study proved otherwise. A group of researchers compared biotin levels in vegans (people who eat no animal products), ovolactovegetarians (people who eat eggs and dairy products), and people who eat a mixed diet. The researchers had logically assumed that biotin levels would be low in vegans and higher in the other groups. But they were surprised to learn that vegans had the highest levels. Two possible explanations were offered. First, the form of biotin found in plant foods may be the most easily absorbed. Second, vegetarian diets may do a better job of helping intestinal bacteria manufacture ample biotin.

Rating: ★

CHOLINE

Present in all living cells, choline is a sort of stepchild in the vitamin B-complex family—technically related but not really a B-vitamin (although it sometimes takes the B-vitamin name). Nonetheless, it has some very important duties in the body. Choline is synthesized from two amino acids, methionine and serine, with help from vitamin B_{12} and folic acid. Choline works together with another lipotropic, inositol, to prevent fat from building up in the liver and to shuttle fat into cells to be burned for energy.

One of the richest sources of choline is lecithin, a fat found in cells and nerve membranes; in egg yolks, soybeans, and corn; and as an essential constituent of animal and vegetable cells. Lecithin helps process cholesterol in the body.

Being so high in choline, lecithin has been dubbed a fat-burner and is available supplementally in capsules, granules, and liquid form. But there's no proof that it helps you burn fat. Lecithin is a fat, and like a fat it provides 9 calories per gram, or 252 calories per ounce. In fact, research shows that a side effect of supplementing with high doses of lecithin is weight gain.

Back to choline. Choline is very important to brain chemistry. In the brain, choline converts to the acetylcholine, a neurotransmitter that sends messages from nerves to nerves and nerves to muscles. When muscles tire out during exercise, this transmission system gets blocked. No messages are sent, and muscle work slows down or ceases temporarily.

Researchers at MIT studied runners before and after the Boston Marathon and found a 40 percent drop in their choline concentrations. They don't know why this happened; however, they speculated that choline is used up during exercise to produce acetylcholine. Once choline is depleted, there's a corresponding drop in acetylcholine production. When production falls off, the ability to do muscle work falls off, too. Theoretically, by supplementing with extra choline, you could work out harder and burn more fat as a result. Of course, we need more research on this issue.

Choline has recently been recognized as an essential nutrient. The National Academy of Sciences has set the RDA for choline as 500 mg for adult men and 425 mg for adult women.

Your body can easily manufacture enough choline for good health as long as you eat a balanced, nutrient-rich diet. Choline is found in eggs, fish, soybeans, liver, brewer's yeast, and wheat germ.

But getting choline from food alone may have a drawback, particularly if you want to keep your brain supplied with choline. Choline is one of the few nutrients that can penetrate the blood-brain barrier, which protects the brain from toxins and other unwanted visitors. Channels to the brain, however, are like limited-access highways where nutrients have to compete for entry like cars trying to get on a road. After you eat a meal (eggs, for example), the choline and amino acids in that meal compete with each other for access to the brain. If you take choline alone—as a supplement—it has no competition and has a direct route to the brain. This is why some nutritionists recommend choline supplementation. To strengthen its effect, try taking choline with water or juice, apart from regular meals.

Rating: ★

INOSITOL

Inositol is rather like choline's twin, meaning that it performs many of the same jobs. It, too, is a stepchild, not considered a full-fledged member of the B-complex family.

Inositol is involved primarily in making lecithin so that fat metabolism can proceed normally. Working together with choline, inositol helps prevent dangerous buildups of fat in the arteries and keeps the liver, heart, and kidneys healthy. Inositol is also helpful in brain cell chemistry, and in high doses (12 to 18 grams a day) appears to be effective in treating depression (12 grams a day) and obsessive-compulsive disorder (18 grams a day).

You also need inositol for the normal functioning of other body cells. This nutrient is required by cells in the bone marrow, eye membranes, and intestines for proper growth.

Your body can make inositol from glucose (blood sugar), and the nutrient is plentiful in whole grains. There is more inositol in the body than any other vitamin, with the exception of the B-vitamin niacin. Too much coffee can deplete your body's reservoir of inositol. This nutrient is available from whole grains, citrus fruits, brewer's yeast, and liver. You get about a gram of inositol daily from food.

Rating: ★

LIPOIC ACID (ALPHA LIPOIC ACID)

At the nutritional center stage of late is lipoic acid (also called alpha lipoic acid), once thought to be a member of the B-complex family. Like choline and inositol, it is now considered a nonvitamin because the body can make enough on its own to prevent a deficiency. Lipoic acid is also available from foods such as potatoes and red meat. But being a "nonvitamin" doesn't mean it's a no-name in nutrition. On the contrary, lipoic acid is getting to be quite a big name.

Like a traffic cop at the cellular level, lipoic acid directs calories from fats and carbohydrates into energy production and away from fat production. More specifically, it is involved in breaking down fats and carbohydrates into fatty acids and blood sugar so they can be converted into fuel for energy. Thus, lipoic acid is a key factor in metabolism.

Lipoic acid's potential value in weight control was discovered in studies of diabetics. Used therapeutically in Germany for more than 30 years to treat diabetes, lipoic acid is a potent weapon against the disease—for two reasons. Reason 1: It normalizes blood sugar by converting it into energy. Reason 2: It helps reduce some of the damage that diabetes can cause—damage to the retina, nerves, and heart.

In studies of diabetics, it was discovered that lipoic acid increases the amount of blood sugar that is changed into energy, without increasing the amount changed into fat. This finding has two important, related implications if you're trying to lose fat or control your weight. First of all, lipoic acid puts the metabolic brakes on fat production, so more of what you eat is burned off as fuel and less is stored as body fat. Of course, supplementing with lipoic acid isn't a license to eat whatever you please. Excess calories—those over and above what your body can burn off—will wind up as body fat. Second—this is key if you exercise—since lipoic acid appears to help your body produce more energy, you should be able to work out harder and longer. A more intense effort helps you develop body-firming muscle (which revs up your metabolism), plus it encourages your body to burn more fat. Lipoic acid can thus help you improve your physique.

There are other reasons besides weight control to consider using lipoic acid. One of its main talents is as an antioxidant to protect the body against disease. In your body is a whole brigade of "terminators" known as antioxidant nutrients: vitamin C, vitamin E, and beta carotene. They actively terminate cellular mischief makers known as free radicals, which were discussed in chapter 1. In the process of terminating free radicals, antioxidants are often temporarily wounded. However, they can be regenerated to their original form by other antioxidants. Lipoic acid is an antioxidant with the power to revamp other antioxidants.

In addition, lipoic acid is a terminator itself. It terminates a free radical known as the hydroxyl radical, which happens to be the most damaging to the body. Lipoic acid also helps produce glutathione in cells. Glutathione is an important antioxidant that regenerates immune cells, prevents cholesterol from becoming toxic, and deactivates cancer-causing substances.

Lipoic acid performs other feats as well. It prevents a protein complex from activating genes that cause cancer, detoxifies the body of metal pollutants, and may retard the progression of HIV infection to full-blown AIDS.

Lipoic acid dwindles as we age, so what we get from food may not be enough. Lipoic acid supplements are sold in health food stores and are definitely worth a look for protecting health. Medical experts recommend taking 20 mg to 50 mg a day as a preventive measure against disease. Based on decades of animal and human research, lipoic acid is safe, even at doses as high as 300 mg to 600 mg a day (the levels used for more than 30 years to treat diabetics). As with any supplement, pregnant women or people with an existing disease should not take lipoic acid except under medical supervision. Lipoic acid may interfere with the body's use of thiamine, so alcoholics or anyone deficient in thiamine should take thiamine supplements while taking lipoic acid.

Lipoic acid leaves the body very quickly. Take it with meals to conserve its use and harness as much of its protective power as possible.

Rating: ★★

GENERAL USE OF LIPOTROPICS

Lipotropics are usually taken with meals. As for exact dosage, it is best to follow the manufacturer's recommendation.

SAFETY CONSIDERATIONS

Generally, most lipotropics are considered safe if not taken in large doses. Very high doses can cause nausea and diarrhea. The levels included in lipotropic formulas do not cause these side effects, however. You can take B-complex lipotropics with other natural weight-loss supplements.

A red flag: Some lipotropic formulations list an ingredient known as ma huang on their labels. Ma huang is another name for ephedra, a short-acting stimulant with potentially lethal side effects. Ephedra can stimulate the central nervous system, causing sleeplessness, anxiety, and nervousness. In susceptible individuals, it can make the heart race and blood pressure soar. Because of these adverse effects, people with heart conditions, high blood pressure, or diabetes should avoid any product containing ma huang. (For more information on ephedra, see chapter 13.)

WHAT'S THE DIFFERENCE BETWEEN A "LIPOTROPIC" AND A "THERMOACTIVE"?

Both are terms used to describe various natural substances promoted for fat-loss, but they do not mean the same thing. "Lipotropic" refers to any nutrient that helps the body utilize fat properly. This involves preventing too much fat from being stored in the liver, aiding in the digestion and absorption of dietary fat, and breaking up cholesterol (a type of fat) so that it can pass through artery walls.

"Thermoactive," on the other hand, is used to describe substances that enhance thermogenesis—the body's production of heat. There are two forms of thermogenesis. One is a release of heat from the burning of food after you eat a meal. The body heats up for a little while, then returns to normal temperature. A supplement that has been found to increase this form of thermogenesis is MCT oil. (For more information on MCT oil, see chapter 8.)

The other form has to do with brown fat, the tissue that specializes in converting energy to heat. As explained earlier, white fat cells store energy in fat's chemical bonds; brown fat cells break apart those bonds and release their stored energy as heat. Another way to put it: Brown fat is the fat that burns white fat. Thermoactive substances are those that theoretically increase brown fat activity. The more active your brown fat, the better you can metabolize stored fat. The only natural substance believed conclusively to activate brown fat is the stimulant ephedra. As previously noted, it has harmful side effects. Other natural substances such as chromium may stimulate brown fat activity, too.

A chemical cousin to ephedra is citrus aurantium, also known as orange bitter oil or synephrine. It may be thermoactive, too, but no one has fully substantiated this effect. If you read that a weight-loss product contains "thermoactives," scrutinize the label. It probably contains ephedra. If it doesn't, then the manufacturer is using the term "thermoactive" loosely. (For more on ephedra and citrus aurantium, see chapter 13.)

FAT-BINDING FIBERS

There's an incredibly easy, no-willpower way to manage your weight—one that most of us should be doing but aren't: eating more fiber. More fiber in your diet will help transform your dieting efforts into something so simple and automatic. You'll be able to keep your weight under control, without even working at it or making yourself crazy.

Fiber (also called roughage) is the nondigestible portion of plant foods. There are two types, soluble and insoluble. Soluble fiber turns into a gel when mixed with water. Good sources include rice, corn, oats, legumes, apples, pears, citrus fruits, bananas, carrots, prunes, cranberries, and seeds. Insoluble fiber absorbs water like a sponge. Examples of foods rich in insoluble fiber include root and leafy vegetables, whole grains, legumes, unpeeled apples, pears, and strawberries.

Dietary fiber has an impressive list of health benefits (see table 5.1), plus several main talents when it comes to weight control.

- **Fiber fills you up but not out.** Soluble fiber, in particular, slows the passage of food from the stomach to the small intestine. This tends to make you feel full after eating. One of the best high-fiber filler-up foods you can eat is oatmeal, according to an Australian study. Bran and other high-fiber cereals aren't bad, either. In a study conducted at the Veterans' Administration Center in Minneapolis, people who feasted on high-fiber cereal for breakfast ate 150 to 200 fewer calories at lunch, compared with those who had low-fiber breakfasts.

Another high-fiber heavyweight is the insoluble fiber pectin—plentiful in apples, oranges, bananas, beets, carrots, and potatoes. Pectin inflates after soaking up water in the stomach, making you feel full.

- **Fiber promotes satiety.** It takes longer to crunch down on and chew up fibrous foods, so your meals last longer. That's a plus, since it takes about twenty minutes after starting a meal for your body to send signals that it's full. With enough fiber at mealtime, you're less likely to stuff yourself and eat too many calories. Besides, fibrous foods add very few calories to your meals.

· **Fiber controls fat and sugar intake.** Fiber-rich diets tend to be low in fat-forming foods such as fats and sugar. By filling up on wholesome, fibrous foods, you have less room for foods that contribute to fat gain.

· **Fiber has a fat-binding effect.** Although fiber slows down the digestion of protein and carbohydrates, it does not do the same with fat. In the digestive system, some fibers naturally bind to fats you eat and help escort them from the body. The net effect is a reduction in the calories left to be stored as body fat.

· **Fiber helps regulate blood sugar.** High-fiber foods require prolonged breakdown, and thus release blood sugar more slowly. This action helps prevent dips in blood sugar—dips that can lead to food cravings. A high-fiber diet helps maintain even energy levels through-out the day.

SCIENTIFIC PROOF

The merits of fiber in controlling weight have been well documented. Study after study shows that people lose weight when they eat more fiber, even if they don't make huge changes in their eating habits.

In a study in Utah, for example, researchers recruited 203 healthy men, aged 21 to 71 years. The subjects ate a diet that was compositionally similar to the average Western diet—roughly 45 percent of total calories from carbohydrates, 16 percent from protein, 36 percent from fat, and 3 percent from alcohol. The researchers wanted to find out how dietary fat, carbohydrate, and fiber were related to body fat percentage. Of all the nutrients studied, fiber had the strongest correlation to body fat. The fattest men in the experimental group ate much less fiber than those with more moderate or low body fat. The researchers recommended that anyone wanting to lose or maintain weight should eat more foods rich in complex carbohydrates and fiber.

Similarly, researchers at the University of Kentucky asked people to consume high-fiber oat bran muffins or cooked beans in their diets—but without making any other dietary changes. The simple addition of extra fiber resulted in 2.2 pounds lost over a 3 week period—automatically and without dieting.

Adding just 7 grams of extra fiber daily can pay off, too. In a 6-month French study, overweight men and women were fed tablets providing 7 grams of beet, barley, and citrus fiber. Part of the group received a placebo, and both groups followed an individualized low-calorie diet. The participants were weighed monthly and periodically evaluated on their level of hunger.

By the end of the experimental period, both groups had lost weight. But the fiber-supplemented participants lost more (over 12 pounds on average, compared with 6.6 pounds in the placebo group). Further, the fiber group felt less hungry during the experiment. The researchers concluded that adding a fiber supplement was of definite value in enhancing weight loss and curbing hunger.

This study brings up a question that begs to be answered: Should you use a fiber supplement to encourage weight loss?

Rule of thumb: Fiber supplements should never replace high-fiber foods. It is always preferable to increase your fiber naturally through eating fiber-rich foods. To get the protective benefits from fiber, the National Research Council recommends eating 20 to 35 grams of fiber a day, both soluble and insoluble. Most people get only about 11 grams a day, however. (For a list of high-fiber foods, see table 5.2.)

Some fiber supplements promoted for weight loss have a troubled past. Take guar gum, for example. In 1990, the FDA halted distribution of one diet product containing this fiber because of reports it can obstruct the throat and because advertising claims for weight loss were unfounded. In fact, between 1972 and 1990, 199 cases of throat obstruction and eight cases of asphyxia (interruption of breathing) were reported. One person died of a blood clot in the lungs after surgery to remove the throat obstruction. (Guar gum is used today mostly as a thickener and food additive in small amounts, uses that do not pose a health risk.)

Several types of fiber are sold in supplement form and may be of some help in managing weight, but only after you have revamped your diet to include more high-fiber choices. A danger with any fiber supplement is abuse through intentional overdosing, especially since fiber supplements are laxatives. Laxative abuse damages the nerves responsible for the colonic contractions that move waste products out of the body. The colon becomes immobilized while the laxatives do all the work. Before long, the colon is impaired, and restoration of normal functioning can take a while. Laxative abuse can also cause potassium depletion.

What follows is a rundown of fibers found in fiber supplements, as well as natural weight-loss supplements, along with their risks and precautions.

CHITIN (CHITOSAN)

What It Is

Chitin, also known as chitosan, is an animal fiber derived from the outer shells of crab and shrimp. It is a waste product of the crabbing and shrimping industry that is also used to make glucosamine, a popular natural remedy for arthritis. As a natural weight-loss supplement, chitin is marketed as a "fat-binder," meaning that it prevents fat absorption in the stomach by attracting fat and entrapping its molecules. This makes the fat molecules too large to be absorbed through the walls of the gastrointestinal tract. As a result, they are excreted from the bowels without being completely digested. By reducing the amount of fat absorbed by the body, chitin theoretically helps in weight control.

Fact and Fiction

Available in Europe for several years, chitin has been tested mostly in animals, where it has been found to lower blood sugar, cholesterol, and triglycerides. Other animal tests indicate that it can help heal wounds and protect cells from environmental pollutants. One company selling the product claims on its Internet web site that in a human study, the average weight loss was 14 pounds in 4 weeks. Also noted were drops in blood pressure, cholesterol, and triglycerides, and an increase in HDL cholesterol.

And, in a Japanese study, eight healthy males who ate chitin biscuits for 14 days (about 3 to 6 grams of chitin daily) experienced significant drops in total cholesterol.

You may find chitin combined with other natural weight-loss substances. One of these is a product called BioZan®, which has been tested in humans. BioZan® contains chitin, oat bran, aloe, beta glucan, and betaine HCL. Oat bran is a fiber known to lower cholesterol, and aloe is an herb with laxative properties. Beta glucan and betaine are both lipotropics, meaning they promote the liver's excretion of fat. (For more information on lipotropics, see chapter 4.)

In a 12-day study in which subjects took BioZan® or a placebo, researchers analyzed the supplement's fat-binding capacity by measuring the amount of fat in stool samples collected after 24 hours. Follow-up samples were collected on days 10, 11, and 12. By day 12, BioZan® had demonstrated a 63.78 percent increased fat-binding capacity. In other words, more fat was excreted than was absorbed among those taking BioZan®. By forming an insoluble gel, BioZan® traps a significant portion of fat and thus helps usher it through the digestive system and out of the body.

Chitin has also been used in conjunction with an herbal supplement called hydroxycitric acid (HCA) and chromium to produce weight loss. In an Italian study, 150 obese subjects were given either the supplement combination or a placebo. Those taking the supplement reduced their weight by 12.5 percent, compared with 4.3 percent among those taking the placebo. Plus, the supplement takers reduced their LDL cholesterol by 35 percent and raised their HDL cholesterol by 14 percent.

Depending on the manufacturer's suggestions, you generally take chitin with water at lunch and dinner.

Safety Considerations

While chitin ushers fat from your body, it may also interfere with the absorption of important nutrients, vitamins A, D, E, and K. Known as the fat-soluble vitamins, these nutrients require fat in order to be transported and used in the body. They have life-supporting functions in the body. By blocking their absorption, chitin could contribute to deficiencies of these essential vitamins. Chitin products typically state this precaution on their labels. Also, chitin was found to decrease calcium absorption in one rat study. Potentially, it could do the same in humans. You should probably avoid chitin if you're trying to increase your calcium intake for health reasons or to prevent osteoporosis.

If you take nutritional supplements such as vitamins and minerals, do not supplement with chitin at the same time. Also, most alternative medicine physicians and nutritionists advise using chitin for no more than 2 weeks at a time.

Rating: ★★

KONJAC ROOT (GLUCOMANNAN)
What It Is

Konjac is a plant related to the yam family. Its root yields a fibrous gel called glucomannan, used as the main ingredient of various natural weight-loss products. The konjac root has been popular in Japan for more than 1,000 years to promote regularity.

Glucomannan may aid weight loss in two possible ways—as an appetite controller and as a fat and sugar binder. Taken with or added to water, glucomannan swells to as much as nine times its dry volume. It makes you feel full and keeps you from overeating. And during digestion, glucomannan is thought to surround sugar and fat molecules, thus minimizing their absorption by the body.

Fact and Fiction

Glucomannan has an impressive list of benefits backed up by plenty of research. In an often-cited eight-week study, for example, twenty volunteers took two 50 mg capsules of glucomannan or a placebo with a cup of water within an hour before breakfast, lunch, and dinner. None of the volunteers followed a special diet or engaged in an exercise program. On average, the volunteers who supplemented with glucomannan lost 5.5 pounds and reduced their LDL cholesterol—all without dieting or exercising. The placebo group lost no weight and experienced no cholesterol-lowering benefits.

Other research shows glucomannan is a well-tolerated remedy for chronic constipation, it reduces unhealthy cholesterol levels, and it helps the body handle glucose better.

Safety Considerations

Because of its binding action, glucomannan may escort valuable nutrients from the body. For this reason, some medical experts say that it should be taken with no more than two meals a day. If you take nutritional supplements such as vitamins and minerals, do not supplement with glucomannan at the same time.

Glucomannan is a very water-soluble fiber. For this reason, be sure to drink plenty of water if you use it. Anyone with swallowing problems or disorders of the esophagus should not take glucomannan—or any other fiber supplement, for that matter. These fibers can potentially expand in the throat and lodge there, causing serious problems.

Rating: ★★

PSYLLIUM

What It Is

Psyllium is a natural bulk-forming laxative made from the seeds of the plantago plant (cultivated in Europe). Found in supplements such as Metamucil, psyllium is a type of soluble fiber known as "hemicellulose," noted for its ability to hold water and form a gel in the stomach. This adds bulk and can make you feel full.

Fact and Fiction

Psyllium is a gentle, effective laxative that passes through the intestinal tract, holding fluids, toxins, and other waste products as it goes. The extra bulk it provides enhances elimination. Studies have shown that it may have a beneficial effect on cholesterol and blood sugar levels. Its bulk-forming ability may help curb your desire to eat. Also, research has found that psyllium does usher some undigested fat from the body.

Although not technically a natural weight-loss supplement, psyllium can give you a sensation of fullness, plus slash your intake of dietary fat. When nondieting volunteers in a London study supplemented with psyllium, they felt much fuller an hour after their meal and ate 15 grams less fat a day than usual.

Another forte of psyllium is its ability to reduce the risk of heart disease by lowering levels of dangerous cholesterol in the body. So solid is the proof behind its cholesterol-lowering effect that the FDA ruled in 1998 that foods containing 2.6 grams per serving of psyllium could be labeled as heart-healthy when consumed as part of a low-fat diet.

Safety Considerations

Some people may be allergic to psyllium. Reactions can range from a mild rash to breathing problems, even death. It may also interfere with the absorption of some vitamins and minerals, so don't take a psyllium supplement at the same time you take a vitamin/mineral pill. Be sure to take psyllium with at least 8 ounces of fluid to prevent possible obstructions in the esophagus or stomach.

Rating: ★★

Table 5.1 Health Benefits of Dietary Fiber

Enhances elimination

Relieves constipation and hemorrhoids

Prevents diverticulosis

Ushers carcinogens from body

Lowers harmful cholesterol and triglycerides, possibly reducing the risk of heart disease

Protects against gallstone formation

Prevents bacterial infection of the appendix

Improves body's handling of blood sugar

Table 5.2 High-Fiber Foods

GRAINS AND CEREALS

Food	Serving Size	Fiber (grams)
All-Bran cereal	1/3 cup	8.5
Barley, cooked	1/2 cup	3.0
Bulgur wheat	1 cup	3.0
Oatmeal, cooked	3/4 cup	1.6
Brown rice	1 cup	1.6
Shredded Wheat	2 biscuits	1
100% stone-ground whole wheat bread	1 slice	less than 1

VEGETABLES

Food	Serving Size	Fiber (grams)
Beans, kidney	3/4 cup	9.3
Beans, garbanzo	1/2 cup	5
Corn	1/2 cup	4.7
Beans, pinto	1/2 cup	4
Potato, baked, with skin	1 medium	4
Peas	1 cup	3.2
Carrots, cooked	1/2 cup	3.2
Beans, lima	1 cup	3
Broccoli	1 cup	2.8
Lentils	1 cup	2.4
Brussels sprouts	1 cup	2.1
Yams	1 cup	1.8
Beans, green, cooked	1 cup	1.2
Spinach	1/2 cup	1

FRUITS

Food	Serving size	Fiber (grams)
Figs, dried	3 medium	7.2
Prunes, dried	3 medium	4.7
Pear	1 medium	4.1
Apple	1 large	4.0
Banana	1 medium	3.8
Blackberries	1/2 cup	3.3
Apple	1 small	2.8
Strawberries	1 cup	2.8
Apricots	3 medium	1.4
Peach	1 medium	1.3

Source: Adapted from *Composition of Foods, Agriculture Handbook no. 8* (Agricultural Research Service, U.S. Department of Agriculture), U.S. Government Printing Office: Washington, D.C., 1975. J. W. Anderson and S. R. Bridges, "Dietary Fiber Content of Selected Foods," *American Journal of Clinical Nutrition* 47 (1988): 440–447; and J. Pennington and H. Church, *Bowes' and Church's Foods Values of Portions Commonly Used*, 14th ed. (Philadelphia: J. B. Lippincott, 1985).

PART II

NATURAL APPETITE SUPPRESSANTS

5-HTP: THE MOOD BOOSTER
THAT HELPS PREVENT WEIGHT GAIN

You know the feeling. You're suddenly overcome by an urge to eat the most fattening foods you can get your hands on: cookies, candy, chocolate, french fries, potato chips, and the like. You succumb, of course; stuff yourself; and then ride out the waves of guilt for being a food weakling. It happens to us all.

What makes us do these things?

In a sense, our ravenous indulgences are "all in our heads." Scientists now know that our desire to eat is not always based on our bodies' actual need for fuel. It may also be based on fluctuating levels of a brain chemical known as serotonin. When its levels dip, hunger sets in, cravings intensify, and we succumb to those cravings. Eating certain foods, particularly sugary ones, increases serotonin and makes us feel better. But alas, we can experience weight gains ranging from 5 to 10 pounds up to full-blown obesity as a consequence of repeated indulgences.

Both of the now-banned weight-loss drugs worked by boosting brain levels of serotonin or by stabilizing its release. Fortunately, there is now an all-natural alternative easily obtainable in health food stores. It is called 5-HTP (5 hydroxy-tryptophan), a naturally occurring compound shown to be effective in the treatment of obesity, depression, anxiety, stress, and other disorders.

WHAT IS 5-HTP?

5-HTP is a chemical cousin to tryptophan, an essential amino acid found in protein. To see how 5-HTP works, it is important to understand more about its relationship to tryptophan and serotonin.

Tryptophan is a precursor, or building block, of 5-HTP, which in turn is ultimately converted to serotonin. Protein foods such as milk and poultry are rich sources of tryptophan. A lack of tryptophan flowing into the brain can result in depression, increased sensitivity to pain, and wakefulness.

You would think that eating a high-protein diet would help deliver more tryptophan to the brain, but this is not so. Protein foods contain other amino acids besides tryptophan, and in larger amounts. To reach the brain, these amino acids must cross the blood-brain barrier, a protective network of tightly knit cells lining the blood vessels of the brain. These cells are trusty, vigilant receptionists who screen substances for entry into the brain and bar the door to unwelcome toxins. Those substances that do get in are ferried across the blood-brain barrier by special carrier molecules. Like a passenger vying for a seat on a crowded bus, tryptophan has to compete with five larger amino acids for a ride over. Consequently, not much tryptophan enters, so very little serotonin is synthesized in the brain in response to a high-protein meal.

However, if carbohydrate foods are eaten with protein foods, the carbohydrate helps deliver more tryptophan to the brain. Carbohydrate triggers the release of the hormone insulin, which drives amino acids into brain cells. Thus, eating high-carbohydrate meals—not high-protein meals—ships tryptophan into the brain, where it can be converted into 5-HTP and eventually into serotonin. This partly explains why high-carbohydrate meals, by raising brain levels of serotonin, satisfy hunger and reduce your urge to overeat. High-carb weight-loss diets are often recommended to treat obesity because serotonin levels in obese patients are sometimes below average. Theoretically, high-carb meals work with your brain chemistry rather than against it.

When you eat mixed meals containing carbs and protein, brain cells take up tryptophan and turn it into 5-HTP, which is then converted into serotonin. Since that's the case, couldn't you just supplement your meals with tryptophan to elevate serotonin in the brain?

No—for several reasons. Less than 1 percent of supplementary tryptophan ever makes it to the brain. Most of it is reshuffled back into making other body proteins, and a good deal is converted into the B-vitamin niacin.

But regardless, tryptophan isn't available as a nutritional supplement anymore, although for years it was very popular. People took it in rather hefty doses (500 mg to 3,000 mg daily) to combat depression, anxiety, premenstrual tension, insomnia, and other ailments. But in 1989, the FDA yanked tryptophan from the market when thousands of Americans developed a crippling illness called eosinophilia-myalgia syndrome after taking tainted tryptophan made by a Japanese chemical company. Although some recovered rapidly after stopping the supplements, thirty-eight people died. Others had lingering damage, including inflammation, muscle pain and fatigue, scarring of connective tissue around muscle, and deterioration of nerves and muscle. Unfortunately, there aren't many effective treatments for this syndrome, particularly in its later stages, and many victims become permanently disabled.

There is still some controversy over whether the contaminated batch was the sole reason for the illness. The FDA believes its investigation of the matter points to multiple factors, including tryptophan itself, as culprits in the outbreak of eosinophilia-myalgia syndrome. Other medical authorities aren't so sure, and assert that overwhelming evidence supports tryptophan's safety.

The supplement 5-HTP is positioned as a safe, natural alternative to both tryptophan and diet drugs such as phen-fen and Redux for elevating serotonin. Studied for more than 25 years, 5-HTP is chemically related to tryptophan but is not the same nutrient. It lies outside the FDA's ban and is considered safe for use. However, the FDA remains suspicious of 5-HTP.

Commercially, 5-HTP is extracted from the bean of Griffonia simplicifolia, a plant native to Africa. Thus, 5-HTP is totally natural. It is not chemically synthesized or produced by bacterial fermentation (as was the suspect, contaminated tryptophan). About the size of a coffee bean, Griffonia is also used in the pharmaceutical production of natural compounds called lectins, which have important medical applications.

Natural 5-HTP appears to work better than tryptophan ever did at increasing serotonin. 5-HTP is ten times more active than tryptophan and easily crosses the blood-brain barrier intact. Unlike tryptophan, it doesn't have to be converted to the B-vitamin niacin. 5-HTP's ability to support serotonin production and naturally boost its levels has made it a potentially effective addition to natural weight-loss supplements. You can find it in tablets and special drink mixes.

Some formulations combine 5-HTP with St. John's wort, a herb known to relieve depression naturally. In scientific circles, it is believed that St. John's wort works by slowing the breakdown of serotonin, thus stabilizing its levels. To my knowledge, however, no tests have been conducted on the effectiveness of combining 5-HTP with St. John's wort to promote weight loss.

Herbs such as the stimulant yerba maté may be paired with 5-HTP. (Refer to chapter 13 for important safety information on diet herbs.)

HOW 5-HTP WORKS

5-HTP May Promote Weight Loss Without Dieting

It's every dieter's dream: slimming down without starving. In several clinical trials, dosages of between 600 mg and 900 mg of 5-HTP led to weight losses averaging 3.1 to 3.7 pounds over periods of 5 to 6 weeks. At first glance, that may seem like an insignificant amount of weight—until you consider that the losses were achieved *without dieting.*

5-HTP Helps You Stick to Your Diet

If you do cut calories, then 5-HTP may help you stay the course. When diets restricted to 1,200 calories daily were combined with supplementation, weight loss was greater—between 6.8 and 7.3 pounds over 5 to 6 weeks.

There's a possibility that supplementing with 5-HTP could help you avoid the mental slumps that often accompany dieting. Research indicates that during a diet, mental function becomes impaired, attention span is shortened, and reaction time is slower. No one knows for sure whether these side effects of dieting are a result of low serotonin or of a change in eating habits. But if low serotonin is the problem, 5-HTP could certainly help you stay mentally alert and active during a diet—and potentially be more motivated to stick with it.

5-HTP Cuts Your Urge to Overeat

5-HTP doesn't have any direct effect on fat-burning, but it does suppress the appetite and makes you eat less, with or without dieting. The reason for this is that 5-HTP naturally elevates concentrations of serotonin in the brain. This reduces your desire to eat. Further, it curtails your craving for carbohydrates—a finding that was observed in the weight-loss studies. Eating fewer carbohydrates is known to help your body enter a fat-burning mode. By reducing your carbohydrate consumption, you inhibit the release of the insulin. This in turn stimulates another hormone, glucagon, which helps unlock fat stores so that they can be burned for energy.

OTHER REMARKABLE HEALTH BENEFITS

5-HTP Treats Depression and Its Symptoms

Most of the excitement over 5-HTP has been generated by its effectiveness in treating depression. Depression affects one out of every four people, according to most reports. It is an emotional disorder with a wide range of symptoms, including withdrawal, inactivity, feelings of helplessness, and anxiety. Low levels of serotonin are thought to be associated with depression. A study conducted in Switzerland found that 5-HTP works as well as the antidepressant fluvoxamine in reducing the symptoms of depression but is better tolerated and has fewer side effects.

Additionally, 5-HTP has been found to reduce anxiety and provide relief to patients suffering from panic disorder.

5-HTP Helps Relieve Migraine Headaches

Approximately 42 million people suffer from headaches, including tension and migraine headaches. Migraines are characterized by intense, gripping pain that may throb. They are sometimes accompanied by nausea and vomiting. A growing body of research has found that migraines originate within the brain and may involve serotonin levels. In Spain, researchers compared the effects of 5-HTP with those of the headache drug methysergide maleate (Sansert) and found that 5-HTP worked as well, with fewer side effects.

5-HTP May Improve Sleep

Researchers who study the lifestyles of people who stay healthy well into their golden years have identified a number of health habits shared by the fit. One of these is sleeping 7 to 8 hours a night. Sleep revives you mentally and physically. It improves your productivity and creativity, and restores your brain function, including information-processing. During sleep, the repair of all body tissues takes place, and disease-fighting systems are bolstered.

Health experts believe that sleep deprivation has become one of the most pervasive health problems in the United States, responsible for personality disorders, traffic accidents, debilitating fatigue, memory loss, decreased physical performance, and illness.

Thus, many curatives for sleep problems have been sought. One might prove to be 5-HTP. When taken on an empty stomach an hour before bedtime, 100 mg of 5-HTP may have the ability to send you into a sound sleep, according to some preliminary research. The reason for this apparent benefit is that 5-HTP, along with tryptophan, is used to make melatonin, a hormone produced by the pineal gland, which is located in the middle of the brain. Melatonin's job is to set and regulate the internal clock that controls the body's natural rhythms. Before any definitive conclusions can be drawn, however, additional research is needed to learn more about 5-HTP's effect on sleep patterns.

HOW TO USE 5-HTP

Worth noting is that the dosages used in the initial studies were very high, and thus not too affordable or practical for the average person.

However, some medical authorities feel that smaller doses of 5-HTP may enhance the effectiveness of other natural weight-loss supplements—which is why 5-HTP is combined in diet aids with appetite-suppressing amino acids. Also, in smaller doses 5-HTP helps reduce stress and depression—both of which can lead to overeating. (For more information on natural supplements that combat stress, see chapter 12.)

Researchers who have studied 5-HTP feel that the supplement works well as an appetite suppressant at relatively low doses—50 mg to 100 mg daily, taken 30 minutes before meals. Supplement manufacturers may suggest other dosages, depending on how they formulate their products.

5-HTP AND DIET

If you don't like to diet—and who does?—then you might try supplementing with 5-HTP and not worrying about cutting calories. Don't go hog-wild, however, by gorging on ice cream, pizza, candy, and other sugary, fatty foods. Just try to make healthier food choices by following the guidelines in appendix A. A well-balanced diet of adequate protein and carbohydrates is best.

Also, vitamin B_6 (pyridoxine), which is plentiful in meats and whole grains, is required by the enzyme involved in the conversion of 5-HTP to serotonin. You need a minimum of 10 mg of vitamin B_6 daily to facilitate the conversion. This amount can be easily obtained from food and a regular multivitamin pill. If you supplement with vitamins, take your pill at least 6 hours before taking 5-HTP, to make sure vitamin B_6 is properly distributed in your body.

Interestingly, eating ten bananas will elevate serotonin concentrations in the blood as much as 100 mg of 5-HTP will. Bananas are high in serotonin, but eating too many is certainly counterproductive to weight loss.

SAFETY CONSIDERATIONS

In larger doses (starting at 200 mg), there can be side effects in sensitive people. These may include stomach upset, constipation, headache, and sinus problems. Lower doses, as recommended above, produce few side effects and potentially help alleviate the underlying emotional causes of overeating.

Among natural weight-loss supplements, 5-HTP seems to have the most contraindications—conditions that make supplementation inadvisable. What's more, the FDA is fearful that 5-HTP could lead to some of the health problems seen with tryptophan. Here are some important guidelines.

· Alcohol affects the metabolism of 5-HTP, so avoid drinking alcohol while supplementing. You should forgo alcohol when trying to shed fat, anyway. Alcohol is a carbohydrate, but it's not first converted to glucose, as other carbohydrates are. Instead, it is transformed into fatty acids, and thus is more likely to be stored as body fat. So if you drink, alcohol puts fat-burning on hold. It's not a dieter's friend!

· Do not supplement with 5-HTP if you're at risk of heart disease or stroke or have high blood pressure, since serotonin is involved in the constriction of blood vessels and blood clotting.

· Do not take 5-HTP if you're using other medications that affect serotonin levels. These include anti-depressants, such as monoamine oxidase inhibitors and Prozac, or prescription weight-loss drugs.

Get your physician's blessing before supplementing with 5-HTP, particularly if you have any preexisting medical conditions.

Rating: ★

SEVEN

AMINO ACID THERAPY: STOP FOOD CRAVINGS

Want to tame a roaring appetite? Try amino acids. By definition, amino acids are linked pieces of protein that we get from food or that our bodies make on their own. Individual amino acids are isolated and produced as "free-form" amino acid supplements. You can purchase them as capsules, in powdered nutritional drinks, or in sports nutrition bars.

Amino acids have far-reaching duties in the body—from building and repairing tissue to producing chemicals that make our brains function. Numbering twenty-two in all, amino acids are divided into two groups: essential, or indispensable, amino acids and dispensable, or nonessential, amino acids. Essential amino acids cannot be manufactured by the body, or are manufactured in very small amounts. You have to get them from protein foods and combinations of vegetable foods. Your body continually takes apart amino acids in foods and then uses them to create new protein—in your blood, in your hair and fingernails, and in your muscles. In fact, your body cannot manufacture protein unless all of the essential amino acids are present. There are nine essential amino acids: histidine, isoleucine, leucine, lysine, methionine, phenylalanine, threonine, tryptophan, and valine.

As for nonessential amino acids, your body can make them by itself from vitamins and other amino acids. The term "nonessential" is somewhat of a misnomer, though, since all amino acids are essential to proper metabolism. Plus, nonessential amino acids become very essential during sickness and stress. The thirteen nonessential amino acids are alanine, arginine, aspargine, aspartic acid, cysteine, cystine, glutamic acid, glutamine, glycine, hydroxyproline, proline, serine, and tyrosine.

Supplemental amino acids have become popular for a wide range of uses, some backed by solid research, others by flimsy claims. One of the most intriguing applications of amino acid supplementation is appetite suppression. Taken in supplemental form, amino acids naturally stimulate and elevate body chemicals that curb appetite. With your appetite under better control, you're less likely to succumb to food cravings and sudden urges to overeat. Still other amino acids appear to be involved in the release of hormones responsible for lean body weight. Here's a rundown on the amino acids most frequently used for weight control and some examples of their risks and benefits.

PHENYLALANINE

Phenylalanine, an essential amino acid, is a building block for certain brain neurotransmitters. Neurotransmitters are chemical messengers that relay information between the brain and the rest of the nervous system. This amino acid has sometimes been used to treat depression because it provides an amphetamine-like boost in mood. Since many people overeat when depressed, phenylalanine's anti-depression properties are beneficial for maintaining a positive mental attitude while dieting. The amino acid is also believed to have a favorable effect on memory and alertness. Because of its ability to preserve endorphins (the body's natural painkillers), phenylalanine has been used for pain relief and the treatment of arthritis.

For weight loss and management, phenylalanine naturally controls food cravings and suppresses your appetite—in several ways. Phenylalanine

- Aids in the natural production of two brain chemicals, norepineph-rine and dopamine, which help control appetite and elevate mood

- Boosts the production of a hormone called cholecystokinin, which may send "stop-eating" signals to the brain. The hypothalamus and the stomach both release cholecystokinin

- Assists in the production of the thyroid hormone thyroxin, which controls the rate at which we burn fat

- May fight chocolate cravings. Some nutritional scientists believe chocolate cravings are related to a deficiency of phenylalanine. Chocolate contains phenylalanine, which may be responsible for the temporary high you get after satisfying your craving.

Phenylalanine is found naturally in almonds, avocados, bananas, cheese, cottage cheese, nonfat dried milk, chocolate, pumpkin seeds, and sesame seeds.

How to Use It

This supplement is usually found as dl-phenylalanine. To reduce hunger, phenylalanine (500 to 1,000 mg) can be taken with water 30 minutes before a meal. Vitamin C and vitamin B_6 are required for the conversion of phenylalanine into neurotransmitters. Thus, supplementing with both vitamins is often recommended when taking phenylalanine.

Safety Considerations

Phenylalanine should be avoided by anyone taking anti-depressants; suffering from high blood pressure, the genetic illness phenylketonuria (PKU), diabetes, or migraine headaches; or being treated for melanoma, a serious form of skin cancer. The supplement could aggravate these conditions. You shouldn't supplement with isolated amino acids for longer than a few weeks.

Rating: ★★

TYROSINE

Tyrosine is made from phenylalanine and is therefore considered a nonessential amino acid. Nonetheless, it has a number of vital tasks in the body. Tyrosine is involved in the formation of red and white blood cells; plays an important role in the activities of the adrenal, pituitary, and thyroid glands; and, like phenylalanine, is a building block of the appetite-suppressing neurotransmitters norepinephrine and dopamine. Also like phenylalanine, tryosine has been used to relieve depression and increase mental alertness.

Tyrosine also boosts the body's production of the hormone adrenaline (also known as epinephrine). Among other functions, one of adrenaline's jobs is to increase fatty acids in the bloodstream so that your body can use them for fuel.

Tyrosine is found naturally in almonds, avocados, bananas, cheese, lima beans, and pumpkin seeds.

How to Take It

Used as an appetite suppressant, tyrosine can be taken before meals in doses of 250 mg or 500 mg each time. Vitamins C and vitamins B_6 are involved in converting tyrosine into neurotransmitters, so supplementing with these vitamins is often recommended. Tryosine should not be taken with a supplement of valine, another amino acid. Valine may bar tyrosine's entry into the brain.

Safety Considerations

Do not supplement with tyrosine if you're taking beta-blocker drugs or anti-depressants, or suffering from high blood pressure (tyrosine may cause blood pressure to rise even higher). If you're allergic to any foods containing tyrosine, do not supplement. Because tyrosine is so closely related to phenylalanine, the same cautions apply.

Additionally, you shouldn't supplement with isolated amino acids for longer than a few weeks.

Rating: ★★

METHIONINE

An ingredient in many lipotropic (fat-mobilizing) supplements, methionine has been linked to weight control. In a number of studies, overweight people who supplemented with methionine and phenylalanine were able to curb their appetites significantly—and lose weight in the process. In combination with phenylalanine, methionine apparently assists in the breakdown of fat.

Rich food sources of methionine include eggs, fish, meat, and milk. There is no appreciable amount of methionine in plant foods.

How to Use It

Using between 500 mg and 1 gram of methionine daily may be helpful in breaking down fat and suppressing your appetite.

Safety Considerations

Methionine can be taken safely by most people. There are some exceptions, however. If you have high cholesterol or a family history of cholesterol problems, avoid methionine. It is involved in the production of homocysteine, a proteinlike substance found in the tissues and blood. High homocysteine levels have been linked to cholesterol formation and heart disease. Paradoxically, however, methionine may help rid the body of fatty substances that clog the arteries.

There are no known interactions between methionine and medicines or other nutritional supplements.

You shouldn't supplement with isolated amino acids for longer than a few weeks.

Rating: ★

GLUTAMINE

Glutamine is the amino acid of the moment; that is, it has been in the nutritional spotlight because of its amazing versatility. Glutamine is the most abundant amino acid in your body. Most of it is stored in your muscles, although rather significant amounts are found in your brain, lungs, blood, and liver. It serves as a building block for proteins, nucleotides (structural units of RNA and DNA), and other amino acids, and is the principal fuel source for cells that make up your immune system.

There was a time when glutamine was thought to be a nonessential amino acid, but now it has been rechristened "conditionally essential." This means you need it when you're ill, stressed, or recovering from surgery. During such times, the demand for glutamine exceeds its production and the body's nitrogen stores become rapidly depleted—a sign that muscle protein is being broken down.

This is a problem, since glutamine is required for healing internal tissues and manufacturing muscle protein. Patients hospitalized for surgery, trauma, or infection often receive supplemental glutamine in their feeding solutions.

Glutamine is depleted during a different kind of stress, too: intense exercise. A group of researchers measured plasma levels of glutamine in runners following their participation in a marathon. For about an hour after the event, glutamine levels declined, then slowly returned to normal within about 16 hours of the race. During this period, the runners' lymphocyte (white blood cell) count declined. Interestingly, lymphocytes rely on glutamine for growth.

In a separate study by the same group of researchers, athletes supplemented with 5 grams of glutamine right after exercise and again 2 hours later. Only 19 percent of the glutamine-supplemented athletes reported infections during the next week, while 51 percent of those who took a placebo got a cold or other infection. Studies like this one have led researchers to believe that the increased incidence of colds, infections, and other illnesses among athletes after intense exercise sessions may have something to do with a glutamine/lymphocyte connection.

But is glutamine a bona fide weight-loss aid?

Recent studies reveal that supplementing with glutamine can curb the desire for sugary foods—an excess of which leads to fat gain. Additionally, glutamine naturally elevates levels of growth hormone in the body. Growth hormone is a substance that makes cells multiply faster. Among other functions, growth hormone helps mobilize fat from storage and makes more fat available for energy. It also promotes the transport of certain essential amino acids inside muscle cells to stimulate muscle growth. For these reasons, growth hormone may be one of the most important hormones for dieters and exercisers because of its powerful actions in fat-burning and muscle-building.

In a study at Louisiana State University College of Medicine in Shreveport, researchers found that oral supplementation with glutamine dramatically elevated growth-hormone levels. Nine healthy volunteers (ages 32 to 64 years) were given 2 grams of glutamine over a 20-minute period, 45 minutes following breakfast. Blood samples taken every half-hour over 90 minutes revealed a 430 percent hike in growth-hormone levels. Theoretically, supplementing with glutamine may help you build and maintain fat-burning muscle tissue, particularly if you exercise regularly.

How to Use It

Between 200 mg and 1 gram of glutamine can be taken with water 30 minutes before meals to lessen the desire for sugary foods and to stimulate growth-hormone release. Both heat and acid destroy glutamine, so you should not take it with hot or acidic foods, such as vinegar.

Safety Considerations

Patients with liver or kidney disease should not supplement with glutamine because it can aggravate these conditions and interfere with their treatment. Glutamine safety studies have been conducted using healthy volunteers who took doses of 0.75 grams per 2.2 lbs (1 kg) of body weight. No side effects occurred at those doses.

To be on the safe side, you shouldn't supplement with isolated amino acids for longer than a few weeks.

Rating: ★★

GROWTH-HORMONE RELEASERS

A trio of amino acids—arginine, ornithine, and lysine—is reputed to work as a "growth-hormone releaser," and thus to be able to help the body build muscle and burn fat. But there's not much research in this area, and what little there is, disproves this claim.

When injected into the bloodstream, arginine does stimulate the release of growth hormone. In fact, arginine injections have been used to detect growth-hormone deficiencies in children.

The most often cited study supporting the growth-hormone releaser theory is one in which fifteen healthy men, aged 15 to 20 years, were given arginine, lysine, or a combination of both on an empty stomach. Levels of growth hormone were measured at four 30-minute intervals after the amino acids were taken. Arginine or lysine given alone produced only slight increases, but when 1,200 mg of each were taken together, growth hormone was significantly elevated—7.3 times higher than what lysine did alone and ten times higher than what arginine produced alone. The age of the participants in this study has to be taken into consideration. Most were in their teens, when growth hormone tends to be more active. By contrast, a similar combination of arginine and lysine given to healthy older men had a minimal effect on growth-hormone release, according to a 1993 study. It's well established that our natural levels of growth hormone start dropping off after age thirty—which may partly explain why we start to gain weight in all the wrong places as we age.

Ornithine, a nonessential amino acid made from arginine, is thought to be an even more powerful growth-hormone releaser. But again, the evidence is lacking. In one series of experiments, subjects took arginine and ornithine in oral doses of up to 20 grams a day. There was hardly any effect, even when supplementers participated in a strength-training program (strength-training boosts the release of growth hormone). Taking the ornithine/arginine duo at bedtime has been often recommended because it supposedly boosts the metabolism more efficiently at night. There's no evidence backing up this claim, however.

These three amino acids are notable for other duties. Arginine is considered a nonessential amino acid, meaning the body can synthesize it from proteins and other nutrients. Meat, poultry, and fish are good sources. Despite the fact that arginine is labeled nonessential, it has a number of important functions in the body. It is essential for growing children and is needed supplementally by people with liver or kidney disease. Arginine is also required to manufacture creatine, an important chemical in the muscles that provides the energy for contractions.

Arginine apparently helps to prevent the body from breaking down protein in muscles and organs to repair itself when injured. In one study, surgical patients who were given 15 grams of arginine daily following their operations had a 60 percent reduction in protein loss compared with non-supplemented patients. Of course, more studies are needed in this area, and you shouldn't self-medicate with arginine, or any other amino acid, after you've been injured unless you have your doctor's permission.

Foods rich in arginine include brown rice, nuts, seeds, oatmeal, cereals, raisins, and whole-wheat products.

Ornithine helps deliver fat to the liver to be broken down. It thus prevents fatty buildup in the liver.

Lysine is an essential amino acid that aids in the absorption of calcium from food and is involved in the formation of the matrix of bone, cartilage, and connective tissue. It is involved in the formation of muscle as well. Lysine also acts as an antioxidant that attacks disease-causing free radicals.

Much has been made of lysine as a natural remedy for cold sores, shingles, and genital herpes. In the 1950s, researchers discovered that the herpes virus can't survive without a supply of arginine. Lysine competes with arginine, muscling it out of the way and making it unavailable to the herpes virus. Theoretically, lysine prevents the multiplication of the virus and staves off a full-blown infection.

Dairy products, fish, lima beans, soy products, and potatoes are all high in lysine.

How to Use Them

Like most amino acids, growth-hormone releasers require no digestion and thus can be taken on an empty stomach, with water or a little fruit juice. Follow the manufacturer's recommendations for usage.

Safety Considerations

None of these amino acids should be taken if you are pregnant or nursing, or have any disease, unless you first get the blessing of your doctor. Taking arginine or ornithine can aggravate herpes.

You shouldn't supplement with isolated amino acids for longer than a few weeks. Long-term use of any amino acid supplement can hurt you. Excess amino acids in your system increase the formation of urea and other wastes. Overproduction of urea leads to gout, loss of calcium, and potential kidney problems because the kidneys have to work extra hard to turn urea into urine and excrete it.

Rating: ★

COMBINATION AMINO ACID SUPPLEMENTS

On health food store and pharmacy shelves, you'll find natural weight-loss supplements that are formulated with combinations of amino acids. One of the more popular is a product called Phen-Cal™, manufactured by Schiff®, a Weider Nutritional International Company. It contains 2,700 mg of dl-phenylalanine, 300 mg of tyrosine, 150 mg of glutamine, 15 mg of 5-HTP (see chapter 6), 30 mg of vitamin B$_6$ (see chapter 4), 200 mcg of chromium picolinate (see chapter 3), and 60 mg of carnitine (see chapter 2). Users are instructed to take six tablets a day.

PhenCal has a fascinating history. It was first developed in the 1980s as a potential treatment for alcohol and drug addiction, and was found to be effective. The reason? Its ability to stimulate the release of dopamine. Dopamine is a pleasure-producing neurotransmitter; at high levels in the brain, it makes you feel good.

It has been theorized that cocaine and other addictive drugs produce their high by stimulating the production of dopamine in the pleasure centers of the brain. However, continued use of these drugs tends to dull dopamine receptors on nerve cells. In other words, cells don't recognize or use dopamine properly. The addict doesn't feel satisfied, and so larger doses of the drug are needed to produce the high, which is really a dopamine burst.

Through a series of biochemical reactions, the body can convert the amino acids—tyrosine, in particular—into dopamine and other brain chemicals. Experiments have shown that supplementing with amino acids reduces cravings for drugs and eases withdrawal symptoms considerably.

Sweets, carbohydrates, and alcohol also stimulate the release of dopamine to varying degrees. But by giving the brain a burst of dopamine through amino acid supplementation, food cravings are cut off at the pass—which is the whole idea behind PhenCal. The supplement supplies the brain with the amino acid building blocks it needs to manufacture and release dopamine naturally.

PhenCal was launched as a natural weight-loss aid in June 1997 and racked up $2 million in sales in its first two weeks on the shelves. The manufacturers have tested its effectiveness in two separate studies. In the first one, overweight volunteers supplemented with PhenCal while following a controlled diet and exercise program. They lost an average of 27 pounds in 90 days. Could this weight loss have been due to the other ingredients in PhenCal, such as carnitine or chromium picolinate? Possibly. But the second study sheds more light on why the supplement seems to be effective at promoting weight loss.

This study, which lasted two years, measured PhenCal's effect on food binges among 130 volunteers. Prior to supplementing with PhenCal, the subjects averaged about twelve binges a week. After being treated with PhenCal, they reduced their number of binges by 73 percent (just under four binges a week)—even while following a low-calorie diet and participating in an exercise program. The results of both experiments are quite impressive. The point is that PhenCal may exert its weight-loss effect by curbing cravings and keeping a raging appetite at bay. Also, no significant side effects have been reported with PhenCal supplementation.

THE HYPE OVER HYDROXYPROLINE

One of the hottest natural weight-loss products being sold currently has liquid collagen as its principal ingredient. Collagen is the major structural protein found in connective tissues such as cartilage, ligaments, skin, and bones. The primary constituent of collagen is the nonessential amino acid hydroxyproline.

This collagen-containing product was first developed in Canada as a feed for chickens. After it was discovered that the chickens gained lean mass, the product was turned into a weight-loss aid for people and sold through a network marketing system. The product also contains aloe vera, a potent laxative.

Reports of its success by users are dramatic and compelling, and many health-care practitioners, including physicians, have been promoting it. The product claims to support lean muscle mass and facilitate fat loss. Some people lose weight on it; others do not. Interestingly, there's a recommended diet to follow while supplementing. But if you stuck to the diet alone, you'd naturally lose weight, whether supplementing or not. Many people who have tried the supplement say it tastes like liquid plastic.

There is absolutely no scientific support for the use of liquid collagen or hydroxyproline for weight loss. Supplementing with this product supplies only a very incomplete source of protein and nothing else. Incidentally, gelatin also happens to be collagen. If you want to supplement with liquid collagen for some reason, simply drink gelatin dissolved in juice.

This current fad is a repackaging of the liquid protein diets popular in the 1970s but no longer recommended. The only difference is that with the current product you are instructed to follow a diet, while the liquid protein diet was used as a meal substitute supplying only about 400 calories a day. By the end of 1977, thousands of people had gone on this unsafe and overly restrictive diet. As reported to the Centers for Disease Control, sixty people died as a result of ventricular arrhythmias (irregular heartbeat). The liquid protein diet, probably because it resulted in the loss of heart muscle, was implicated as the cause of the fatal heart problems.

PART III

NATURAL METABOLIC BOOSTERS

EIGHT

MCT OIL: KICK-START YOUR METABOLISM WITH THIS "FATLESS" FAT

Think about it: Whenever you've embarked on a weight-loss diet, one of the first recommendations you've always heard was to "cut the fat." But what if you were told to "up the fat"? Without feeling guilty, you can do just that—as long as that fat is MCT oil, short for "medium-chain triglycerides."

WHAT IS MCT OIL?

MCT oil is a special type of dietary fat that was first formulated in the 1950s by the pharmaceutical industry for patients who had trouble digesting regular fats. It is processed mainly from coconut oil but does not seem to have any of the adverse side effects associated with tropical oils, such as elevated LDL cholesterol. MCT oils occurs naturally in many of the foods we eat and is quite plentiful in human milk. Still used in medical settings as part of feeding formulas for critically ill patients, MCT oil is available in health food stores as a nutritional supplement that aids in weight loss and helps boost energy.

MCT oil is no ordinary fat. Although it tastes much like regular salad oil, that's where the similarities end. At the molecular level, MCT oil is structured very differently from conventional fats such as butter, margarine, and vegetable oil. This structure gives it some unique properties. To understand them, let's first look at the differences between conventional fats and MCT oil.

Conventional fats and body fat are made up of long carbon chains, with sixteen or more carbon atoms strung together, and are thus known as long-chain triglycerides or LCTs. MCT oil, on the other hand, has a much shorter carbon chain of only six to twelve carbon atoms—thus, it is called a medium-chain triglyceride. These molecular differences cause MCTs and LCTs to be used quite differently by the body.

To be digested, LCTs must first be broken down in the watery medium of the intestines. This is an elaborate process because LCTs, like most oils, do not dissolve in water by themselves. They require bile salts, which are secreted by the gallbladder. In a process called emulsification, a molecule of bile acid attaches itself to a molecule of fat, dispersing the fat into the watery solution where it can meet an enzyme. A similar reaction occurs when you wash clothes. The laundry detergent acts as an emulsifier to dissolve the grease, molecule by molecule, suspending it in water so that it can be rinsed away.

Enzymes break the fat down into fatty acids, which then cross the membrane of the intestine and are resynthesized into fats. The newly re-formed fats combine with a special type of protein so that they can be picked up by the lymphatic system and carried to the liver (the primary site of metabolism) for further processing. From there, the fat is released into the bloodstream, where it is picked up by fat cells and eventually stored as body fat if not used immediately for energy. But because the body prefers to use glucose and amino acids first, LCTs tend to be stored as body fat.

Fewer reactions are involved in the digestion and absorption of MCTs. Because of its shorter chain, MCT oil is metabolized much more quickly than fatty acids from regular oils or fats.

Unlike LCTs, MCTs are more water-soluble. They can be absorbed more easily through the intestinal wall, requiring fewer enzymes or bile salts. An enzyme in the intestinal wall breaks MCTs down into fatty fragments that combine with a water-soluble protein in the blood. From there, MCTs go right into the bloodstream and are transported to the liver, where, inside the cells, they are rapidly oxidized or burned up.

HOW MCT OIL WORKS

MCT Oil Is Generally Not Stored as Body Fat

MCT oil is burned up so quickly that its calories are turned into body heat—a process known as thermogenesis, which boosts the metabolic rate. The higher your metabolism, the more calories your body burns.

Several studies in animals and humans have tested MCT oil's thermogenic effect. An often-cited study that looked into this effect was published in the journal *Metabolism* in 1989. To determine whether MCT oil affected thermogenesis differently than regular fats, ten men (ages 22 to 44 years) were fed liquid diets containing 40 percent of fat in the form of either MCTs or regular fats. After 5 days on this diet, thermogenesis increased significantly in the men who consumed MCTs—but remained unchanged in the men who ate regular fats. The researchers concluded that MCT oil stimulated thermogenesis better than an equivalent amount of conventional fat did. They also noted that MCT oil was less likely to be stored, compared with other fats.

More recently, a 1996 study found that because MCT oil is so readily metabolized—whereas conventional fat is not—weight gain is minimized with the addition of MCT oil to the diet.

Basically, very little of this remarkable fat leaves the liver; therefore, MCTs rarely end up being stored as body fat—a scenario that does not occur with conventional fats. So by using MCT oil, you can have your fat and eat it, too, because it is immediately burned for energy and therefore is not stored as body fat, like conventional fats and oils.

MCT Oil Boosts Your Metabolism

Because MCT oil is thermogenic (heat-producing), it can rev up the metabolism—which potentially means you can burn more fat. Researchers at the University of Rochester looked into this possibility. In an experiment involving seven healthy men, they tested whether a single meal of MCTs would increase the metabolic rate more than an LCT meal would. The men ate test meals containing 48 grams of MCT oil or 45 grams of corn oil, given in random order on separate days.

In the study, metabolic rate increased 12 percent over 6 hours after the men ate the MCT meals but increased only 4 percent after LCTs were consumed. What's more, concentrations of fats in plasma (the liquid portion of blood) were elevated 68 percent after the LCT meal but did not change after the MCT meal. These findings led the researchers to speculate that replacing LCTs with MCTs over a long period of time might be beneficial in weight loss.

MCT Oil Maximizes Your Calorie-Burning Potential

To a certain extent, losing fat depends on energy balance, a kind of biological banking system your body uses to maintain its weight. You deposit energy in the form of calories from food and then withdraw, or spend, that energy to live, breathe, move, and exercise. As long as your deposits equal your expenditures, your body generally maintains its weight.

But if you deposit more calories than your body can spend, you can gain fat. To lose it, you have to create a calorie deficit by eating less, exercising more, or both. Now, according to a recent scientific study, there's another way to get that deficit—without sweating or depriving yourself—by supplementing with MCT oil.

When eight healthy men at the University of Geneva took just 1 to 2 tablespoons of MCT oil as part of their daily normal diet, their daily caloric expenditure increased by 5 percent! On average, they burned 113 extra calories a day.

What does this mean to you? Suppose, for example, you're eating roughly 2,000 calories a day, with part of those calories coming from MCT oil. You'd effortlessly spend an additional 100 calories a day—the equivalent of walking for 30 minutes at a moderate pace. You'd burn extra calories, without any extra effort!

MCT Oil Spares Protein

A healthy goal of any fat-loss program is to preserve as much muscle tissue as possible. The more muscle you have, the better your body can burn fat. This is because muscle is the body's most metabolically active tissue. It burns calories even at rest. Fat tissue is not as active.

Unfortunately, far too many diets overrestrict calories. Severe caloric restriction forces the body to start cannibalizing its own precious muscle tissue (including heart tissue) for energy.

You can guard your muscle by following a calorie-adequate diet, sticking to an exercise program that includes strength-training—and supplementing with MCT oil. In a study at Calgary University in Canada, healthy adults were placed on a low-carbohydrate diet supplemented with MCT oil. The researchers measured the use of fat and protein in the subjects' bodies and found that there was an increase in body fat burned and a decrease in muscle protein used for energy. In other words, MCTs helped burn fat and, at the same time, preserved lean muscle by preventing its breakdown.

MCT Oil Increases Endurance

Exercise is an important way to encourage fat loss. The harder and longer you exercise, the more fat you can burn. But often, it's tough to exercise all-out, and one reason is low energy. That's where MCT oil can help.

First, it provides twice the energy of protein and carbohydrates (8.3 calories per gram versus 4 calories per gram for carbohydrates and protein), and is absorbed into the bloodstream as rapidly as glucose, the cellular fuel made available from the breakdown of carbohydrates.

Second, MCT oil is preferentially used as fuel for energy, instead of being stored by the body. Medium-chain fatty acid fragments can diffuse very quickly into the cell, where they are burned immediately for energy—at the same time as glucose. The ability of MCTs to enter the cells in this manner has a glucose-sparing effect, meaning that glucose and its stored counterpart, muscle glycogen, last longer without being depleted. The longer glycogen reserves last, the more energy you have for activities and fat-burning exercise.

To boost your endurance during exercise, take MCT oil with a carbohydrate source such as a sports drink. At the University of Capetown Medical School in South Africa, researchers mixed 86 grams of MCT oil (nearly 3 tablespoons) with 2 liters of 10 percent glucose drink to see what effect it would have on the performance of six endurance-trained cyclists. The cyclists were fed a drink consisting of glucose alone, glucose plus MCT oil, or MCT oil alone. In the laboratory, they pedaled at moderate intensity for about 2 hours and then completed a higher-intensity time trial. They performed this cycling routine on three separate occasions, so that each cyclist used each type of drink once. The cyclists sipped the drink every 10 minutes. Performance improved the most when the cyclists supplemented with the MCT/glucose mixture. The researchers did some further biochemical tests on the cyclists and confirmed that the combination spared glycogen while making fat more accessible for fuel.

MCT Oil Can Replace Some of Your Carbohydrate Fuel for Faster Fat-Burning

Carbohydrates such as rice, cereal, pasta, breads, fruits, potatoes, and sweet potatoes offer a mother lode of vital nutrients. But too much carbohydrate in your diet can be fat-forming, particularly if you're not very active. A carbohydrate overload triggers a surge of insulin into your bloodstream. Insulin activates enzymes that move fat from the bloodstream into fat cells for storage, and this action spells extra weight for many of us.

When you reduce your intake of carbohydrates, you suppress the release of insulin. Low insulin stimulates the release of another hormone, glucagon. As glucagon goes to work, it signals the body to start burning fat for energy.

Reducing carbohydrate intake to lose weight has long been the basis of many diets. And for good reason—it works. But there are penalties. Carbohydrate is your body's leading nutrient fuel. During digestion, carbohydrate is broken down into glucose. Glucose circulates in the blood to be used for energy. If your muscles are deprived of glucose, your physical power suffers. You're low on gas, and feel it. It becomes tough to stick to your eating program, and another attempt to lose weight could bite the dust.

But MCT oil can come to the rescue. You can still apply the low-carb dieting strategy, but without the corresponding loss of energy! Remember:

MCT oil is burned in the body like a carbohydrate and spares glucose fuel for an energy-boosting effect.

Thus, by supplementing with MCT oil, you have a pure energy source to help prevent diet-induced fatigue. At the same time, MCT oil keeps your metabolism high, and a high metabolism is conducive to losing body fat.

How, then, should you plan your weight-loss diet to take advantage of MCT oil's power? What follows is a sample diet plan that will show you how to substitute MCT oil for high-starch foods to facilitate fat-burning.

THE MCT OIL DIET

This diet consists of 20 to 30 percent protein, 50 to 60 percent carbohydrates, and the rest from fat, including MCT oil. Along with the restriction of carbohydrates, the higher percentage of protein in the diet helps control hormones (less insulin, more glucagon) in favor of fat loss. Carbohydrates, however, are plentiful at breakfast, midmorning snack-time, and lunch to provide adequate fuel for the day's activities. But carbs are limited at night—when they are less likely to be fully burned through exercise or activity. Below is a template to help you plan your daily menu:

Breakfast

> 1 serving (1/2 cup) of a whole-grain cereal
> 1 cup nonfat milk
> 1 serving of a lean protein (such as 4 to 6 egg
>   whites or a protein powder shake)
> 1 serving fruit

Midmorning Snack

> 1 serving fresh fruit or a sports nutrition bar

Lunch

> 3 ounces lean protein source, such as turkey, fish, or lean red meat
> 1 cup cooked nonstarchy vegetable (salad vegetables, broccoli, cauliflower,
>   green beans, carrots, spinach or other green leafy vegetable, and so forth)
> 4 ounces starchy vegetable (baked potato, brown rice, yams, or legumes), 2
>   teaspoons margarine or conventional vegetable oil

Midafternoon Snack

> 8 ounces plain nonfat yogurt, sweetened with artificial sweetener or 2
>   teaspoons low-sugar jam; sports nutrition bar; or fresh fruit

Dinner

> 3 ounces lean protein source, such as turkey, chicken, or lean red meat
> Liberal amounts of nonstarchy vegetables, such as a large salad of chopped raw vegetables
> 2–3 tablespoons French dressing made with MCT oil (see recipe on p. 95)

Here's what a day's menu might look like:

Breakfast

> 1/2 cup Bran Buds cereal
> 1 cup nonfat milk
> 4 scrambled egg whites
> 1 cup melon balls

Midmorning Snack

> 1 medium apple

Lunch

> 3 ounces baked chicken breast
> 1 cup cooked broccoli
> 4 ounces baked potato topped with 2 teaspoons margarine

Midafternoon Snack

> 8 ounces plain nonfat yogurt, sweetened with artificial sweetener or 2 teaspoons low-sugar jam

Dinner

> 3 ounces baked or grilled salmon
>
> Large salad: 2 cups romaine lettuce, 1 chopped fresh tomato, 4 tablespoons chopped raw onion, 1 chopped carrot
> 2–3 tablespoons French dressing made with MCT oil

The above menu supplies about 1,450 calories; 33 grams of fiber; ample vitamins and minerals (including calcium); and antioxidant nutrients, which protect against disease and bolster immunity.

Excluding carbohydrates after lunch may cause a drop in your energy levels late in the day. Compensate by using MCT oil (up to a tablespoon), taken with some nonstarchy vegetables for an afternoon snack. Used this way, MCT oil moves your body into a fat-burning mode and helps speed up your metabolism.

Stay on a diet plan like this no more than 2 weeks at a time. After 2 weeks, add a serving or two of high-starch carbohydrates, preferably natural ones such as potatoes and whole grains, to your diet. Natural carbohydrates are used more efficiently by the body than their processed counterparts (breads and pastas) because they are preferentially stored as glycogen, rather than as fat, if not used first for energy.

HOW TO USE MCT OIL

MCT oil should always be taken with food, and can be poured over vegetables or made into salad dressings (see the recipes on page 95). You can also cook or bake with MCT oil just as you would with any other vegetable oil. Keep the heat at 350 degrees or lower, however, because MCT oil smokes at high temperatures. Don't store MCT oil in anything other than a glass container. It tends to soften containers made of certain types of plastic.

Gradually introduce MCT oil into your diet at the rate of a few teaspoons a day until you are consuming 2 to 3 tablespoons a day. MCT oil contains 114 calories per tablespoon. This supplement is so rapidly absorbed that it tends to cause stomach cramping if too much is taken at one time or on an empty stomach.

Make sure you purchase pure MCT oil, not a product that's diluted. How can you tell? A good rule of thumb is that any MCT oil product that comes flavored is not the pure stuff. Read the label to see whether the product is cut with flavorings or other fillers.

SAFETY CONSIDERATIONS

MCT oil is generally safe for most people, except those with preexisting medical conditions. The supplement is not advised if you have a fatty liver or cirrhosis, because the fat is channeled directly into an already poorly working liver. Nor should you use MCT oil if you suffer from chronic pulmonary disease such as emphysema or asthma, because it results in greater production of carbon dioxide—a side effect that can further complicate breathing. If you are diabetic, avoid MCT oil, because it promotes the production of toxic substances known as ketones in diabetics.

MCT oil does not supply essential fatty acids (EFAs)—vitamin-like substances that have a protective effect on the body and are necessary for life. The best sources of these healthy fats are olive oil, canola oil, safflower oil, and other vegetable oils. Make sure you're eating at least 2 teaspoons of such fats daily. Never substitute MCT oil entirely for essential fats in your diet. You will risk an essential fatty acid deficiency, which can show up as dry, flaky skin and stiff, painful joints. These symptoms may indicate that your heart, brain, liver, and internal organs are EFA-deficient as well.

Rating: ★★★

MCT OIL RECIPES

FRENCH DRESSING WITH MCT OIL

1/2 cup MCT oil (nonflavored)
1/4 cup red wine vinegar
1 teaspoon salt
1/2 teaspoon dry mustard
1/2 teaspoon paprika

Shake together all ingredients in a tightly covered glass jar; refrigerate. 90 calories per tablespoon.

ITALIAN DRESSING WITH MCT OIL

1 cup MCT oil
1/4 cup vinegar
1 tablespoon finely chopped onion
1 teaspoon salt
1 teaspoon sugar
1 tablespoon Italian spices
2 teaspoons chopped garlic
1/4 teaspoon black pepper

Shake together all ingredients in a tightly covered glass jar; refrigerate. 100 calories per tablespoon.

NINE

CREATINE: THE ENERGIZER THAT HELPS DEVELOP BODY-SHAPING MUSCLE

Attention, exercisers: If you want to develop fat-burning muscle tissue faster, try creatine. It's a nondrug alternative that really works! In fact, creatine is probably the most important natural supplement yet to be discovered for exercisers because of its ability to extend endurance and coax the body into producing hard, firm muscle. Even if you don't exercise, you can still gain a little muscle, but your results will be far better with regular workouts.

WHAT IS CREATINE?

Although it is a relatively new natural supplement, creatine was first discovered in meat by a French scientist in 1832. He named it after the Greek word for flesh (*kreas*). Several years later, another investigator found that wild foxes had ten times more creatine in their muscles than less active, domesticated animals—a clue that physical activity may cause creatine to build up in muscle tissue. As early as 1926, a British medical journal reported that natural creatine might be beneficial for weight gain. Synthetic creatine was first produced in the 1950s by a Waukegan, Illinois, pharmaceutical company. And, reportedly, Soviet athletes began using the substance in the 1960s.

But it wasn't until 1992 that creatine grabbed the limelight, when two researchers in Sweden, Paul Greenhaff and Eric Hultman (who developed carbohydrate-loading for endurance athletes), reported on its beneficial effects on exercise performance.

Creatine is produced naturally in the liver, kidneys, and pancreas—at a rate of about 1 to 2 grams a day—from the amino acids arginine, glycine, and methionine. Most of your body's creatine is delivered to the muscles, heart, and other body cells. Inside muscle cells, creatine helps produce and circulate adenosine triphosphate (ATP), the molecular fuel that powers muscular contractions.

Creatine is found naturally in red meat. About 2 1/2 pounds of raw steak yields roughly the equivalent of a single 5-gram dose of creatine. Few other foods provide as much creatine—one reason why vegetarians are often creatine-deficient. Extensively researched, creatine is available as a powdery nutritional supplement known as creatine monohydrate, synthesized from water and two special kinds of salts in a heating process. It is often an ingredient in tablets, protein powders, meal replacers, and nutrition bars formulated for athletes, and is available in health food stores and sporting goods stores.

Through supplementation, you can build the volume of creatine in your muscle cells. There, creatine increases levels of a high-energy compound called creatine phosphate, which serves as a tiny fuel supply, enough for several seconds of action. In fact, supplementing with 20 to 25 grams of creatine daily increases muscle stores of creatine by 20 to 30 percent, and roughly 20 percent is in the form of creatine phosphate.

Creatine phosphate also allows more rapid production of ATP. The more ATP that is available to muscle cells, the longer, harder, and more powerfully you can work out. Thus, creatine can indirectly help you lose body fat, since longer, more intense workouts help incinerate fat and build lean muscle. The more muscle you have, the more efficient your body is at using energy and burning fat.

Creatine is a wonderful performance enhancer if you engage in short-burst activities such as lifting weights, cycling, rowing, swimming, sprinting, or playing sports like soccer and ice hockey. And, unlike a lot of nutritional supplements, it lives up to its claims. A review article in a noted professional journal, *International Journal of Sport Nutrition*, described creatine thus: "Creatine should not be viewed as another gimmick supplement; its ingestion is a means of providing immediate, significant performance improvements to athletes involved in explosive sports."

So popular is creatine—in 1998 alone, sales were expected to surpass $200 million—that many major sports teams use it, including the San Francisco 49ers, the Portland Sea Dogs, and the Los Angeles Lakers, to name just a few.

HOW CREATINE WORKS

Creatine Is a Muscle-Builder

Properly developed muscle is your body's best friend when it comes to losing fat and maintaining your weight. Remember: Firm, strong muscles are metabolically active. This means they can burn body fat more efficiently than body fat or untoned muscle, even at rest. Plus, toned muscles help define the body, giving you extra curves where you want them. Achieving good muscle tone comes through exercise, particularly strength-developing exercise, supported by good nutrition and dietary supplementation.

Among the supplements with muscle-making power is creatine. It has been shown to help your body manufacture proteins within muscle fibers. Two of these fibers, actin and myosin, are known as contractile proteins. They slide over each other like two pieces of a telescope to cause muscle contractions. When you build muscle through exercise, diet, and assistance from creatine, you're essentially increasing the amount of contractile protein in your muscle fibers. This makes the muscle fibers expand in diameter, get stronger, and generate more force when they contract.

In 1995, researchers in Dallas put eight weight-trained men on 20 grams of creatine daily for 28 days to test their strength gains and ascertain any changes in body composition. By the end of the experiment, the men increased their lifting capability on the bench press by 18 pounds, on average. That's remarkable progress! What's more, the men showed a 2 percent gain in lean muscle.

Creatine supplementation works fast, too—in as little as one week! A 1997 study conducted at the Pennsylvania State University Center for Sports Medicine demonstrated the immediacy of creatine's strength-building, muscle-building power. The researchers recruited fourteen weight-trained men and divided them into a creatine group and a placebo group. Both groups performed bench presses and a jump-squat exercise in three different sessions, each separated by 6 days. Prior to the first session, neither group received any supplementation. During the period leading up to the second session, both groups took placebos. Then, prior to the third session, the creatine group took 25 grams of creatine monohydrate a day, and the placebo group took a 25-gram placebo. All the participants were asked to follow their normal diets and keep food records during the experimental period.

With this well-designed experimental situation, the researchers could easily observe and measure any changes due to supplementation. What happened was quite remarkable. In just a week, the creatine takers gained an average of 3 pounds of weight (one gained nearly 6 pounds). As for their strength, it went through the roof. The creatine takers upped their repetitions significantly on the bench press and could perform more jump-squats. Those in the placebo group didn't fare as well in either performance or body weight gain.

Other creatine supplementation studies have shown gains in body mass averaging 2 to 6 pounds, usually within several weeks of use. It is important to point out that some of the weight gain experienced by creatine users is due to water. Creatine attracts water into the muscle cell, and this action inflates muscles so that they look fuller. Some people like this look, others do not. Still, not all the gain is water. Body composition testing of creatine users has verified that much of the weight gain is lean muscle.

Creatine Boosts Your Energy

Instead of pooping out during workouts, you can keep going with extra creatine loaded into your muscles. The surplus boosts the pace of energy production in the muscle cell and allows the muscle fibers to work harder, longer. In one study, eight physical education students took creatine supplements for 5 days, and another group took placebos. Following the supplementation period, the students exercised on a stationary bicycle, performing 130 pedal revolutions for 10 seconds, interspersed with 30 seconds of rest. The next day, they upped their revolutions to 140 to induce greater fatigue.

Compared with the placebo group, the creatine group could do more revolutions per minute over the final moments of each exercise routine. The placebo group fizzled out much sooner than the creatine group. Clearly, creatine supplementation maximized energy for this type of short-duration activity and postponed fatigue.

In a study of twenty-four competitive rowers, supplementation with 20 grams of creatine for 5 days extended the athletes' rowing time and enabled them to push even harder on the last leg of their race.

By keeping your muscles loaded with creatine, you can head fatigue off at the pass while exercising. Creatine depletion in muscle cells is a major cause of fatigue. The results of research into creatine prove this point. In one study, researchers looked at creatine levels in sprinters and found that their muscle supply fell markedly according to the length of the sprints. After 100 meters, creatine levels dropped by 50 percent; after 200 meters, 59 percent; and after 400 meters, 90 percent. When creatine stores were fully drained, complete fatigue set in.

Creatine May Reduce Muscle "Burn"

As noted earlier, creatine increases concentrations of creatine phosphate in muscle cells. Creatine phosphate interferes with the production of lactic acid, which is a waste product of short-burst exercise that accumulates in the muscles and blood. A buildup of lactic acid is what makes your muscles "burn" after repeated contractions. Too much of this acid in the muscles wears you down while you're working out. By cutting lactic acid levels, you can work out for longer periods of time before tiring out—and burn more fat in the process.

OTHER REMARKABLE HEALTH BENEFITS

Creatine May Favorably Alter Cholesterol and Triglyceride Levels

High concentrations of these fatty substances can contribute to heart disease. At least one study has found that creatine supplementation may reduce their concentrations. A team of researchers in Dallas looked into the effects of a combination of 5 grams of creatine monohydrate and 1 gram of glucose, or a placebo, on the blood chemistry of thirty-four men and women, ages 32 to 70 years. Compared with those given the placebo, the creatine-supplemented group showed marked declines in total cholesterol, triglycerides, and very low-density cholesterol (a particularly dangerous type of cholesterol) after 51 days of supplementation. It's not clear why there was such a positive effect, but creatine certainly looks like a contender as a lipid-lowering agent. Of course, much more research is needed to verify this benefit.

Creatine Helps Treat Diseases

In their excellent book *Creatine: Nature's Muscle Builder*, Ray Sahelian, M.D., and Dave Tuttle report that creatine can be successful against an eye disease called gyrate atrophy that, if untreated, can lead to blindness. The authors also note that creatine may be helpful in treating muscle-wasting caused by AIDS and degenerative diseases.

HOW TO USE CREATINE

Increasing the levels of creatine and creatine phosphate in your muscles gives your working muscles another fuel source besides glycogen from carbohydrates. The question is, how much creatine do you need? You do get creatine from food—roughly 1 gram a day. But you'll need more to enhance your exercise performance and fat-loss efforts. Scientific research shows that taking four 5-gram doses a day (5 grams is about a teaspoon) for 5 days will do the trick. This is known as the "loading phase."

Sports nutritionists recommend matching your dosages to your body weight. If you weigh under 150 pounds, for example, take 10 to 12 grams daily during your loading phase; 150 to 170 pounds, 15 to 20 grams; and over 175 pounds, 20 to 25 grams. From there, 2 to 5 grams once a day—about half a teaspoon—will keep your muscles saturated with enough extra creatine. This period is called the "maintenance phase."

One of the best times to supplement with creatine is right before your workout. That way, you can load it into your muscles at just the right time to start replenishing muscle reserves and restocking ATP. Taking it after your workout is a good idea, too. Creatine enhances the movement of amino acids in cells for tissue growth and repair following exercise.

Pure creatine has no flavor, so you can mix it with plain water, a sports drink, or a noncitrus fruit juice (citrus juices neutralize creatine, and the supplement loses its effect). Nor is coffee a good choice. Research shows that caffeine counteracts creatine and blocks its strength-producing benefits.

Creatine does not dissolve well in fluid. But not to worry, it is absorbed very well by the body. Exciting new research shows that creatine may work best in combination with a liquid carbohydrate supplement. In fact, this combination boosts the amount of creatine accumulated in muscles by as much as 60 percent!

In a recent study, investigators divided twenty-four men (average age was 24 years) into experimental and control groups. The control group took 5 grams of creatine in sugar-free orange juice four times a day for 5 days. The experimental group took the same dose of creatine, followed 30 minutes later by 17 ounces of a solution containing carbs. Muscle biopsies taken following the 5-day test period showed that both groups had elevated creatine levels—but with one dramatic difference. Creatine levels in the experimental group were 60 percent higher than in the control group. There were also higher concentrations of insulin in the muscles of the experimental group.

The implications of this study to strength-trainers, athletes, and exercisers are enormous. Just think: By supplementing with creatine and carbs at the same time, you're supercharging your body. With more creatine in your muscles, you'll have more power to strength-train.

The fact that the creatine/carb combo increases insulin is equally important. Insulin increases the uptake of glucose, which is ultimately stored as glycogen in the liver and muscles for fuel. The more glycogen you can stockpile, the more energy you'll have for exercise. The creatine/carb combo is a bona fide energy booster for all types of exercise activity.

Even if you stop taking creatine, it will remain in your muscle fibers for some time. Creatine begins to empty out over the course of 4 to 8 weeks. Even the creatine you take during a 5-day loading phase stays in your muscles for about a month. Because creatine sticks around for so long, you can go on and off it—a practice known as "cycling." In other words, you do not have to stay on creatine continually.

Creatine supplementation can be expensive, so view it as an investment in a trimmer, more sculpted you. A 20-to-30-gram loading dose can cost about $7.20 a day; a 10-to-15-gram maintenance dose, $3.60 a day.

Also, make sure you purchase creatine from a well-known manufacturer. Some creatine on health food store shelves is impure, reportedly cut with baking soda or contaminated with rat hairs. Apparently, some of the impure stuff has come from China.

CREATINE AND DIET

To support muscle growth, creatine works best with a nutritious diet that supplies ample calories. Figure out your calorie needs, based on your present body weight. Here are some examples:

To build muscle, if you're a man, eat 23 to 27 calories per pound of body weight a day. So if you weigh 165, your caloric range would be 3,795 to 4,455. If you're not yet within range, add calories gradually.

If you're a woman who wants to gain muscle, eat 20 calories per pound of body weight a day. If you weigh 120, you should eat 2,400 calories a day to build muscle.

As you gain muscle, recalculate your calories. Most of your additional calories should come from carbohydrates—in the form of natural, unprocessed food and liquid carbohydrate supplements or sports drinks. Carbs supply the energy to drive the muscle-building process and are critical for replenishing lost glycogen following a hard workout. Approximately 60 to 65 percent of your total daily calories should come from carbohydrates when supplementing with creatine.

Protein intake is critical, too, especially for the repair and construction of muscle tissue following exercise. If you lift weights as part of your muscle-building program, you definitely need more protein. About 15 to 20 percent of total daily calories should come from lean protein. Another way to figure appropriate protein intake is 0.7 gram of protein per pound of body weight daily (slightly more—about 0.9 gram per pound of body weight—if you do aerobics, too). Thus, a strength-training man weighing 165 pounds should eat about 115 grams of protein daily; a 120-pound woman, about 84 grams.

Antioxidants such as beta carotene, vitamin C, vitamin E, and selenium are important, too, since they appear to help tissues recover better and regenerate more quickly following exercise. And the need for B-complex vitamins increases with exercise. A good supplement program for strength-training exercisers is as follows:

Antioxidants (daily): 200 to 300 mg of vitamin C, 100 to 400 IU of vitamin E, 10,000 to 20,00 IU of beta carotene, up to 50 mcg of selenium.

B-complex vitamins: For every 1,000 calories of carbs you consume daily, you need 0.5 mg of thiamin; 0.6 mg of riboflavin; and 6.6 mg of niacin. (An antioxidant multiple containing B-complex vitamins should help meet these needs.)

SAFETY CONSIDERATIONS

Creatine monohydrate is nontoxic, and studies have been unable to find any negative side effects from its usage. But if you take too much at once, you can experience stomach upset.

Creatine was in the news a couple of years ago, following the tragic deaths of three college wrestlers who tried to shed weight rapidly in order to qualify for their weight classes. One of the wrestlers, who attempted to lose 12 pounds in a single day, suffered kidney failure and heart malfunction while wearing a rubber suit during a 2-hour workout in 92-degree temperatures. His body contained high concentrations of creatinine, a component of urine that is a breakdown product of creatine. The finding prompted an investigation by the FDA into the effects of supplemental creatine. The FDA concluded that creatine was not a factor in the deaths.

So what led to this tragedy?

The deaths were most likely caused by the wrestlers' dangerous make-weight practices, including severe dehydration and self-imposed sweating. These practices can create a dangerous condition similar to heat stroke, which elevates the level of the creatine breakdown product creatinine in the body.

Creatine has also been associated with cramping and muscle spasms, according to some athletes' trainers, although they can't prove the problems result from the supplementation. Experts feel that these conditions are probably caused by insufficient water intake. Creatine tends to pull water from other parts of the body into cells, so it's important to drink an additional 8 ounces of water daily—over and above your normal 8 to 10 cups a day.

Creatine supplementation is ill-advised if you have preexisting severe kidney disease (for example, renal dialysis or kidney transplant patients). Thus, people with kidney disease should not supplement with creatine. Always consult your physician before supplementing.

Rating: ★★★

REAL-LIFE RESULTS

Joe E., a 46-year-old president and owner of a marketing communications firm, has used creatine several times—each time with positive results. Joe always followed the recommended loading and maintenance dosages on the product's label. For 5 days, he supplemented with 20 grams of creatine, taken four times a day. During the maintenance phase, he cut back to 10 grams, taken in the morning on an empty stomach and again right before his workout, or in the afternoon.

"I tried to mix it with liquid, but the product I was using didn't dissolve well," he described. "So I'd take a scoop of it in my mouth, then wash it down with either white grape juice or a sports drink." (Both beverages are excellent choices. Creatine is shuttled into muscle cells with help from the hormone insulin. Noncitrus fruit juices and sports drinks contain glucose, which causes a surge in insulin. The net effect is more rapid uptake of creatine by the muscles.)

"Within three days—while still in the loading phase—my energy level was at an all-time high. I was lifting more weight during my strength-training workouts and feeling fully energized for the 2-hour basketball game I play three times a week."

Remarkably, in just 3 weeks, Joe's body weight increased from 170 pounds to 178 pounds. To make sure that weight was mostly muscle, he had his body composition tested. Good news: He had reduced his body fat percentage from 10.2 to 9.4 percent. Vacation snapshots revealed a much-improved, aesthetically sculpted physique.

The only side effect Joe noticed from creatine supplementation was the slight water weight gain many users report. "My muscles continued to be larger than before, but eventually took on a more puffed-up look, rather than a sharp definition."

PART IV

NATURAL HERBS FOR WEIGHT MANAGEMENT

TEN

HCA (HYDROXYCITRIC ACID): CONTROL YOUR APPETITE NATURALLY— AND LOSE FAT, TOO

Among natural weight-loss supplements, hydroxycitric acid (HCA) is the jack-of-all-trades. It promises to curb your appetite, shut off food cravings, block your body's production of fat, speed up calorie-burning, conserve lean muscle, and boost energy. That's a tall order to fill, but if you're among the 95 percent of dieters who have tried to lose weight but have not had lasting success, HCA might be just the solution you've been searching for.

WHAT IS HCA?

Chemically similar to the citric acid found in citrus fruits, HCA is extracted from the rind of a sour fruit known as the Malabar tamarind, which is about the size of an orange. It grows on a tree called *Garcinia cambogia*, native to India and southern Asia. Both the fruit and the rind are common foods in this region; people eat them virtually every day. In India, the dried rind is used to flavor curries and preserve fish.

Because of its astringent and antiseptic properties, the rind has long been considered a medicine in India. People there have used it in gargles and taken it orally for stomach problems. The rind is also brewed into a tea, believed to help alleviate joint problems and bowel irregularities. Veterinarians in India use garcinia cambogia to treat mouth diseases in cattle.

The rind has industrial applications as well. It is used to polish gold and silver, and to help manufacture rubber latex. The wood of the tree is suitable for making posts and splints. Additionally, the seeds of the fruit are a rich source of edible fat, high in oleic acid, the most abundant fatty acid found in nature. Without question, garcinia cambogia is a very versatile plant!

HCA can also be extracted from *Garcinia indica*, grown in India and known as the red mango. Like its cousin garcinia cambogia, garcinia indica is prized both as a culinary spice and as a remedy for various medical conditions, including intestinal problems, skin diseases, and wounds. However, garcinia indica has lower concentrations of HCA than garcinia cambogia.

Commercially available in health food stores and pharmacies, fruit-derived HCA is a common ingredient in many weight-loss products under the trade names Citrin®, Citrin®K (which contains the mineral potassium), and Citrimax™. It is found in tablets, nutrition bars, chewing gum, and tea.

HOW IT WORKS

HCA Prevents the Formation of Fat

The fascinating story of HCA began in 1965, when chemists in India first isolated and identified HCA as the principal acid in garcinia cambogia and garcinia indica. It turned out to be no ordinary ingredient. HCA appeared to keep excess carbohydrates from being converted into fat.

This amazing discovery sparked the interest of Hoffmann-La Roche, a huge pharmaceutical company, which sponsored the early groundbreaking studies on HCA at Brandeis University. Research continued for many years. In test tube studies and animal experiments, researchers found that this natural compound did indeed block fat production—a finding that was observed in rat liver cell cultures and in the livers of live rats that were given HCA orally or by injection.

How does HCA perform this amazing feat? The researchers discovered that HCA short-circuits the action of ATP-citrate lyase, an enzyme involved in the conversion of carbohydrates into fat. After you eat a meal, any carbohydrate not used immediately for energy or stored as glycogen is turned into fat in the liver by ATP-citrate lyase. HCA blocks this enzyme and, in the process, curtails the creation of acetyl coenzyme A, a biochemical factor that provides the building blocks for the production of fat. Thus, with a one-two punch, HCA slows down the fat-making process.

HCA Encourages Fat-Burning

According to investigators who study HCA, the production of new fat accounts for a very small portion of weight gain. One study found that the liver manufactured less than a half a gram of fat per day (that's about an eighth of a teaspoon). Thus, they feel that HCA's greatest potential may lie not just in its ability to block fat formation but also in its ability to enhance fat-burning.

How does HCA stimulate fat-burning? Again, the chain of events involves enzymes. At the cellular level, HCA interferes with the production of yet another enzyme, malonyl coenzyme A, also involved in fat synthesis. When malonyl coenzyme A is in short supply, more fat is burned.

HCA Suppresses the Appetite

Wouldn't it be terrific if you could cut your body's hunger signals off at the pass—and do it naturally, without resorting to dangerous appetite-suppressing drugs? It is possible, thanks to HCA's ability to curb the appetite.

The early research into HCA showed that feeding HCA to test animals prevented weight gain in young, growing rats. The rats tended to eat less—*even those rats whose appetite-control centers in the brain had been surgically removed!* What's more, very little HCA was found in the rats' brains. Based on this finding, the researchers suggested that the appetite-curbing effect of HCA may be centered not in the brain (as it is for many appetite-suppressing drugs) but in the liver.

Why the liver? One of the jobs of the liver is to convert energy-containing nutrients from the food you eat into two storage systems: glycogen (the storage form of carbohydrates) and some fat. Glycogen is stored in the liver and muscles, and is used to supply your body's ongoing energy needs. When required for energy, glycogen can be called out of storage in the liver and disassembled into glucose (blood sugar) to fuel the work of your body's cells.

Like a restaurant customer who tells his server he's had enough to eat, the liver lets the brain know when its glycogen stores are filled to capacity. Messages from receptors (specialized cells connected to nerve fibers) in the liver are relayed to the brain via the vagus nerve, a direct communication route to the brain. Once the brain gets the message, your desire to eat dies down.

So where does HCA fit in? The early studies found that HCA accelerates the production and storage of glycogen. This action stimulates the receptors in the liver to signal the brain that glycogen stores are full. The net effect is appetite suppression.

Another appetite-regulating factor related to the presence of HCA may be in force, too. A greater availability of glycogen helps offset low blood sugar and the cravings usually associated with it.

Much of the research uncovering HCA's ability to block fat formation, stimulate fat-burning, and curb appetite has been done with animals. Studies with rats are one thing, but what about experiments with people like you and me?

The promise of HCA demonstrated in animal experiments naturally led to human studies. In one early study of obese men, a dose of 800 mg daily resulted in an average weight loss of 3.5 pounds in just one week.

More recently, Anthony Conte, M.D., a bariatrician (a physician who specializes in the treatment of obesity and diseases related to it), conducted three clinical evaluations of HCA, which were published in the booklet *Citrin®—The Revolutionary, Herbal Approach to Weight Management.* In each study, participants ate a low-fat, low-sugar, low-sodium diet and were encouraged to follow a sensible daily exercise program such as walking—in addition to supplementation with HCA.

In the first study (conducted in 1991), fifty-four people participated. During an 8-week period, thirty participants took Lipodex-2 (a supplement containing 500 mg of HCA and niacin-bound chromium) three times a day, prior to each meal. The other twenty-four participants took a sugar-pill placebo prior to each meal.

The volunteers who supplemented with Lipodex-2 lost an average of 11.1 pounds per person, while those in the placebo group lost 4.2 pounds per person. Dr. Conte noted that the Lipodex-2 group stuck to their diets better than the placebo group did, and had higher energy levels and diminished cravings for sweets.

Conducted in 1993, the second study (also 8 weeks long) compared the weight loss effects of Actotherm (a supplement not formulated with HCA), combination therapy with Actotherm and Lipotrol (which contains Citrin®, a patented form of HCA), and supplementation with Lipotrol alone. A total of ninety-three people completed the study. Here's the summary of how they fared: Supplementing with Lipotrol alone produced an average weight loss of 11.48 pounds per person (twenty-nine participants); combination therapy (Actotherm and Lipotrol), 9.52 pounds per person (thirty-five participants); and Actotherm, 6.65 pounds per person (twenty-nine subjects).

Conte's third study (conducted in 1994) enlisted seventy-five volunteers (sixty men and fifteen women), ranging in age from 21 to 65 years, and weighing from 135 to 253 pounds. Before each meal, they took a supplement formulated with 250 mg of HCA (Citrin®) and 100 mcg of chromium picolinate. Although the volunteers were reasonably healthy, 74 percent had abnormally high levels of blood fats (cholesterol and triglycerides), and 53 percent were on prescription medications for either elevated blood fats or being overweight.

After 8 weeks on the program, forty-two people who completed the study lost an average of 10.8 pounds per person. Of those volunteers, eleven had marked drops in their cholesterol and triglyceride levels. And in eight cases, blood glucose levels dropped significantly. Conte noted, "It is reasonable to conclude that Citrin® plus chromium picolinate in the doses used in this study and in combination with an appropriate diet and exercise plan can facilitate weight loss."

And that weight loss is often dramatic. Writing in *Medical Hypotheses,* one medical researcher who personally tried HCA noted: "As little as one gram before each meal was extremely effective in reducing my own appetite and weight, and resulted in a definite sustained increase in energy, as well as a weight loss of about one pound per day without dieting."

What this all confirms is that supplementing with HCA, coupled with gentle lifestyle changes, is a viable method for permanent pound-paring. But that's not all. There's more good news about HCA for dieters.

HCA Spares Lean Tissue

A diet that overly restricts calories—say to 1,000 calories daily or below—will most certainly produce weight loss—but the wrong kind. Unfortunately, up to 30 percent of what's lost will be muscle (including heart tissue). Here's why: When deprived of food, the body begins to feed on the protein in the muscles. Because muscle is the body's most metabolically active tissue, depleting it interferes with your ability to burn calories.

The scientific studies conducted with animals revealed that HCA not only enhanced fat-burning but also slowed the rate at which body protein (such as muscle tissue) was used up. In other words, lean tissue was conserved. Exactly why this happens is unclear. But it could have something to do with HCA's ability to accelerate the body's glycogen-making process. With more glycogen available for energy, the body need not tap into its protein reservoir for energy. Of course, studies would be needed to confirm this assumption.

If you do diet and find it necessary to restrict calories, supplementing with HCA may help you minimize the loss of lean muscle—in addition to suppressing your appetite and encouraging your body to burn fat.

HCA Elevates Energy

HCA's glycogen-enhancing effects potentially provide a ready supply of additional energy. Considered a vital fuel for exercise, glycogen supports endurance exercise, strength-training, and other physical activities. It is supplied by the diet in the form of carbohydrates. Exercisers, athletes, and other active people could use HCA to help stay "powered up" for exercise and activity. However promising and reasonable this may sound, studies need to be done to confirm this potential benefit.

OTHER REMARKABLE HEALTH BENEFITS

HCA could be a potential weapon against dangerous blood fats, which are culprits in heart disease. Predictors of heart disease include not-so-favorable profiles of cholesterol in the blood and high triglycerides in the blood. The type of cholesterol deposited on the artery walls is low-density lipoprotein (or LDL) cholesterol. LDLs are known as "bad" cholesterol. The lower your blood values, the better.

High-density lipoprotein (or HDL) cholesterol is heart-protective. It transports cholesterol from your cells to your liver for processing and excretion. HDL is the "good" cholesterol because it doesn't clog arteries. The more in your blood, the better. The general recommendation for adults is to have an LDL level of below 130, an HDL level below 35, and a total cholesterol reading below 200.

Triglycerides are one of the major fats in the blood and the chief form of fat in food. High triglycerides, however, can lead to a potentially harmful overproduction of cholesterol in your body. You should have your triglycerides checked regularly, along with your cholesterol. A desirable reading for triglycerides is below 200.

The animal and human studies conducted with HCA showed that the compound reduces levels of dangerous LDL cholesterol and triglycerides in the body. This is most likely due to its ability to inhibit an enzyme (ATP-citrate lyase) involved in the production of fat. Therefore, HCA may have beneficial action in the prevention and treatment of cardiovascular disease.

HOW TO USE HCA

HCA is typically available in supplements as "standardized garcinia cambogia extract," meaning the product contains a precise dose of the isolated active compound. Standardized extracts are usually high-quality sources.

Many companies manufacture HCA-containing supplements. Despite the fact that Hoffman-La Roche conducted the early animal experiments on HCA, the company could not patent the extract at the time because it was a natural ingredient. (This is one of the major reasons pharmaceutical companies are not in the business of producing natural weight-loss supplements.)

Proper dosage is critical. Research suggests that the appropriate dosage for appetite suppression and weight loss is 500 mg to 1,000 mg daily of the standardized extract, divided into smaller dosages taken two to three times a day. HCA is most effective when taken half an hour to an hour before meals.

Using HCA with other nutrients may provide additional benefits. You will find HCA in formulations with ingredients such as chromium and l-carnitine. There are reasons for this. People who are overweight often have insulin-regulation problems. When insulin is out of whack, the body can go into a fat-producing mode. Oversecretion of insulin can trigger the activity of lipoprotein lipase, the enzyme that tells fat cells to start making fat. Enter chromium, a trace mineral essential for normal sugar and fat metabolism. Chromium helps regulate the function of insulin. By making insulin work better, chromium, in effect, inhibits fat synthesis. (To learn more about chromium, see chapter 3.)

The rationale for adding carnitine to HCA weight-loss formulations is generally based on carnitine's reputation as a potential fat-burner. The two ingredients are believed to work as a team, perhaps encouraging faster fat loss—although no research currently substantiates this theory. (For more information on carnitine, see chapter 2.)

Other ingredients may be part of the formulation, and some may be herbs. (To understand exactly what you're buying, please refer to chapter 13.)

HCA AND DIET

For best results when supplementing with HCA, follow a low-fat, moderate-protein, and moderate-carbohydrate diet. Your caloric range should be between 1,200 and 1,500 calories a day (men can go higher—up to 1,800, particularly if you're active). You could certainly lose weight on a diet in this caloric range without supplementing with HCA. However, the addition of HCA may help you stick to the program better because of its ability to suppress the appetite and its potential to help your body burn fat more efficiently.

No more than 20 percent of those calories should come from fat. Populate your daily diet with high-fiber carbohydrates such as whole grains, raw fruits, and vegetables. (Refer to appendix A for a sample diet.)

Refrain from excess alcohol use (no more than two drinks a day) while supplementing with HCA, since alcohol impedes the benefits of HCA. Drink eight to ten glasses of water daily, and try to get some moderate exercise each day. Walking is an excellent choice.

SAFETY CONSIDERATIONS

For centuries, people of India and southern Asia have eaten the fruit and rind of garcinia cambogia without ill effects. Interestingly, the recommended daily dose of HCA in supplement form is equal to nearly half a fruit rind—the daily quantity often consumed by people in southern Asia. Another plus: Health-care practitioners who recommend HCA feel it is suitable for long-term use (twelve to twenty-four months), particularly for keeping lost pounds off—a major challenge for any dieter.

HCA appears to be a safe, sensible way to manage weight. According to researchers, HCA does not cause insomnia, nervousness, depression, high blood pressure, or rapid heartbeat—side effects often associated with over-the-counter diet aids. People who are sensitive to citrus fruits may experience some stomach irritation when supplementing with HCA since it is similar to the citric acid found in those fruits. However, HCA is formulated with the addition of calcium, which acts as a neutralizer to make it less acidic.

Pregnant or lactating women, or young children should not take HCA. And anyone with diabetes, high blood pressure, or any prolonged illness or preexisting medical condition should consult a physician before supplementing.

Rating: ★★★★★

ELEVEN

GUGGUL: A FAT-CONQUERING BOTANICAL

From the oldest of all medicinal systems, Ayurveda (produced eye-yuhr-VAY-dah), comes one of the newest fat-burners available, guggul, referred to as "gulgulipid" in the scientific literature. It potentially offers an easy, no-willpower way to shed excess weight and even restore youthful curves by helping your body incinerate excess fat and calories throughout the day.

WHAT IS GUGGUL?

Guggul (commiphora mukul) is an extract purified from the sap of a small, thorny tree native to India. For centuries, the resin was used as a folk medicine in India to treat intestinal ailments, urinary problems, rheumatism, and obesity. Its active components are two natural plant steroids known as Z-guggulsterone and E-guggulsterone. Supplements in extract form are usually standardized to contain a minimum of 2.5 percent total guggulsterones.

Guggul is often formulated with other nutrients, including chromium, HCA (see chapter 10), and various herbs.

HOW IT WORKS

Guggul May Be a Fat-Burner

In animal studies conducted more than 30 years ago, a scientist in India discovered that test animals lost weight after being given guggul. This sparked interest in guggul as a fat-loss agent.

How guggul actually works in this regard is unclear, but scientists speculate that it exerts its effect partially through the activity of the thyroid gland. The thyroid gland sets the rate at which the breakdown of food into energy (metabolism) takes place, and secretes various hormones. Guggul appears to spark thyroid activity by increasing levels of these hormones. When thyroid function is revved up, the body's metabolic rate is increased, leading to more efficient fat-burning. It is also believed that guggul may stimulate the activity of brown fat—the fat that burns white fat.

Guggul Helps Recontour Your Physique

One landmark study conducted in 1990 reported "significant weight loss" in research with seventy guggul-supplemented subjects. Also reported were considerable body composition changes, including less fat under the skim and trimmed-down hip and waist circumferences.

Guggul also works well when combined with another Ayurvedic supplement, triphala. Triphala, which means "three fruits," is an herbal preparation consisting of three different plants, amla (*Emblica officinalis*), bibitaki (*Terminalia belerica*), and haritaki (*Terminalia chebula*). It is a laxative and an antioxidant. When forty-eight obese volunteers took 500 mg of guggul and triphala three times a day for 3 months, they shed an average of 18 pounds—all without changing their eating habits. Additionally, their total cholesterol count fell 18 points.

OTHER REMARKABLE HEALTH BENEFITS

Guggul May Be Heart-Healthy

The subject of hundreds of scientific studies, guggul is praised for its ability to support healthy cholesterol levels nutritionally. Studies have found that the supplement is effective and safe for lowering LDL cholesterol and triglyceride levels, while maintaining or improving HDL cholesterol. In fact, it is as effective as the synthetic drug clofibrate, used to treat high cholesterol, but demonstrates better compliance and produces fewer side effects.

Studies using 25 mg of gugulipid taken three times a day have shown that cholesterol levels will drop 14 to 27 percent in 1 to 3 months, while triglyceride levels will fall by 22 to 30 percent. Further, gugulipid has been found to prevent the formation of atherosclerosis (a build-up of fatty deposits), as well as reduce existing deposits.

Guggul appears capable of improving cholesterol and triglyceride profiles, and may even reverse atherosclerosis in the aorta, the main artery from which refreshed blood leaves the left chamber of the heart.

In a study of 200 patients with ischemic heart disease, guggul demonstrated several heart-protective effects: Electrocardiogram patterns were restored to normal, blood fats were significantly reduced, and cardiac irregularities were reduced.

Guggul May Help Treat Acne

Acne can be a chronic problem affecting teenagers and adults alike. It occurs when the hair follicles of the skin become plugged, often leading to infection. In serious cases, the infection responds to treatment with the commonly prescribed antibiotic tetracycline. But this medicine has various side effects, including dizziness, lightheadedness, sore joints, and anemia, and thus should not be taken long-term.

An alternative approach may prove to be supplementation with guggul. In a 1994 study, twenty people with cystic acne (a serious form of the disease) were treated with either 500 mg of tetracycline or 25 mg of guggulsterone. Both regimens were taken twice a day for 3 months. By the end of the study, it was found that guggulsterone was slightly more effective than tetracycline in treating acne. Also, patients with the oiliest complexions responded better to the guggul preparation.

Guggul May Be an Anti-Inflammatory Agent

Inflammation is the body's natural defensive response to infection and certain chronic diseases such as rheumatoid arthritis. Inflammation, however, produces pain, swelling, and often redness—which is why anti-inflammatory drugs such as aspirin and ibuprofen are often recommended to reduce the discomfort. But anti-inflammatory drugs are not without their side effects. The active compounds in guggul, Z-guggulsterone and E-guggulsterone, have been studied in India for their effects on joint diseases and have been found to be virtually free of any adverse side effects.

HOW TO USE IT

Look for products standardized to contain guggulsterones, the active components of the herb. To encourage fat loss, informed health practitioners suggest supplementing with one tablet three times a day. Follow the manufacturer's directions for usage, however, since products may vary.

GUGGUL AND DIET

Because guggul appears to help reduce fat in the blood and tissues, it should work optimally in partnership with a low-fat diet. Loading up on fatty foods would only negate the herb's special benefits. (For help in planning a low-fat diet, see appendix A.)

Also, you may want to glean some dietary advice by exploring the Ayurvedic system of medicine, which is largely based on diet. Along with diet, exercise, and lifestyle management, herbs like guggul and triphala are used in this healing system to help restore balance and well-being.

Ayurveda classifies individuals into three health/body types, governed by controlling principles called Vata, Pitta, and Kapha. According to

Ayruvedic thought, all three intermingle in an individual's constitution to some degree, although a single principle may predominate or be out of balance at any given time. You're considered healthy if all three principles are in equilibrium. Practitioners look at the patient's disposition, habits, and life in general to customize the Ayurvedic treatment accordingly.

Vata involves movement, emotions, breathing, circulation, and the nervous system. When balanced, this principle makes you more alert, energetic, and creative. Out of whack, it causes anxiety, restlessness, constipation, and high blood pressure. To help restore balance, dietary recommendations include eating sweet fruits, cooked vegetables and grains, nuts, natural sweeteners, and dairy products in moderation. Foods to avoid are dried fruits and grains, raw vegetables, and any gas-producing food.

The Pitta principle relates to metabolism, and balance leads to healthy digestion and tranquillity. Out of balance, it manifests as anger, skin problems, and ulcers. Dietary steps include eating sweet fruits, vegetables, all types of beans, and milk-based cheeses; and avoiding sour fruits, pungent vegetables such as onions, nuts, spices, and any fermented dairy products such as yogurt.

Kapha describes attributes such as structure and solidity. Balanced Kapha provides strength, endurance, healthy immunity, and a good disposition. An imbalance can make you overweight and lead to related problems, such as water retention and high cholesterol. Foods to balance Kapha include dry fruits, raw vegetables, dry grains and cereals, spicy foods (thought to help the metabolism), and beans. As for diet, low-fat, low-sugar foods—typical of most reducing diets—is the best course of action. Sweet fruits, nuts, natural sweeteners, dairy products, and oil should be avoided, according to Ayurvedic recommendations.

SAFETY CONSIDERATIONS

Studied scientifically for more than 30 years and used in India for more than 2,500 years, guggul appears to be safe as a dietary supplement. If you are taking cholesterol-lowering medication or other drugs, consult with your physician before supplementing.

Rating: ★★

TWELVE

KAVA KAVA AND ST. JOHN'S WORT: TWO CALMER-DOWNERS THAT EASE EMOTIONAL OVEREATING

Are you eating because something is eating you?

Many people turn to food when stressed out or down in the dumps—a habit that can pile on the pounds unless you get it under control. Eating does ease the tension or lift the depression—but only temporarily. After the binge, you are apt to feel even worse emotionally because you've overindulged. Guilt-ridden, you can slip into a vicious cycle of overeating and negative emotions.

If stress or moods regularly cause you to binge, there are many steps you can take to break the cycle, from stress management to behavioral modification to psychological counseling. Ultimately, you must deal with the root cause of what's eating you. But while you're doing the dealing, there are two amazing herbs that can give you a sense of calm on the stormy seas of stress, anxiety, or depression: kava kava and St. John's wort.

Neither is a metabolic substance that encourages fat loss, but both are being included in weight-loss formulas. Here's why: These herbs have a tranquilizing effect on stress and an uplifting effect on blue moods. Because stress and depression compel many people to overeat, supplementing with either kava kava or St. John's wort may quite possibly keep you from raiding the fridge in times of trouble. For that reason, they can be very helpful agents indeed.

(Note: These supplements are not star-rated because therapeutically they are not used for fat loss, only for emotional disorders.)

WHAT IS KAVA KAVA?

Imagine a safe, natural, nonaddictive substance with the power to calm your body and mind, promote restful sleep, banish a bad mood, relax muscle tension and spasms, and soothe anxiety. Sound too good to be true? Probably—but such a substance really does exist!

Meet kava kava, a remarkable herb you can purchase at any health food store without a doctor's prescription. Kava kava is a relatively new herb to the United States, but not to Germany, where it has been available since 1920. Approximately 350,000 prescriptions for kava kava are written annually in Germany for anxiety-related disorders. Kava kava is truly nature's stress cure—one of the best natural relaxers and tranquilizers around.

A member of the pepper family grown in tropical forests, kava kava has been around for thousands of years in the South Pacific, as part of a fermented drink used in religious and social rites. The explorer Captain James Cook may have been one of the first Westerners to ever try it, and he introduced it to the West after a voyage through the South Pacific from 1768 to 1771. Later, kava kava was given its botanical name, *Piper methysticum*, which translated means "intoxicating pepper," reflecting its kinship to the pepper family and its physical effect on the body (*methys* is the Greek word for "drunken"). It is believed to have been first cultivated on the volcanically formed islands of Vanuatu (formerly New Hebrides), where much of it is grown today.

In folk medicine, kava kava has been used to treat kidney and bladder ailments, joint problems, respiratory disorders, stomachaches, backaches, and headaches. It is actually the root of the plant that is used for medicinal purposes. Each year in Europe, 100 tons of the herb are processed into medicinal remedies. Today, kava kava is fast becoming one of the hottest-selling herbs, part of the $12.4 billion+ herb market worldwide.

HOW IT WORKS

Kava kava's therapeutic effects are due to at least fifteen different biological compounds, collectively known as kavapyrones or kavalactones. All are physiologically active, and six are psychoactive. Most of these produce physical and mental relaxation without causing addiction or harmful side effects.

The first kavapyrone was isolated in 1889. Since then, much research has been devoted to identifying the effects of the herb's other kavapyrones. It is now well documented that kavapyrones can alter brain activity without causing sedation, and work as general relaxants, muscle relaxants, local aesthetics, and anti-convulsives.

In 1990, Commission E, Germany's equivalent of our FDA, approved kava kava for treating anxiety, stress, and restlessness. Several well-designed studies conducted in the past ten years support its effectiveness. For example, in 1997, 101 patients suffering from anxiety were given kava

kava over the course of a 25-week double-blind study. By the eighth week, anxiety symptoms in those taking kava kava had subsided considerably, compared with those given a placebo. The researchers noted that kava kava is an effective, well-tolerated alternative to drugs commonly used to treat anxiety and depression.

There are times, however, when prescription drugs are necessary, and chances are, your physician or psychiatrist will prescribe them. But before you swallow another drug with side effects that could harm you, understand what it does and how it might affect you. Of course, some of these drugs are less than ideal. Many can dull your senses and be addictive. Other side effects include nausea, bloating, abdominal cramping, and dizziness. By contrast, kava kava leaves your mental sharpness intact, is not habit-forming, and imparts a sense of tranquillity without the worrisome side effects of prescription medications.

Kava kava helps you manage stress in two important ways. First, it counteracts the physical symptoms of stress, such as pounding heartbeat or tensed muscles. Second, it works on brain chemicals to produce a calming effect, as well as on regions of the brain responsible for emotion.

Kava kava is fast-acting, too, providing relief within about half an hour to two hours. Although known best for its tranquilizing ability, kava kava also contains two pain-relieving chemicals (dihydrokavain, and dihydromethysticin) that are as effective as aspirin.

Worth noting, too, is that kava kava is believed to be thermogenic; that is, it may increase body temperature and thus burn additional calories. The herb has been used in some parts of the world as a weight-loss agent.

In many cases of stress and emotional disorders, kava kava should be the first choice in treatment because it works with your body rather than against it.

HOW TO USE IT

Kava kava is available in several forms: capsules, liquids, bulk, teas, standardized extracts, single-herb, and multiherb. As for supplementation, a good rule of thumb is to abide by the manufacturer's recommended dosage or by Commission E's recommendations of daily dosages of 60 to 120 mg of kavapyrones or kavalactones. Make sure to purchase a product that is standardized to contain kavapyrones or kavalactones.

SAFETY CONSIDERATIONS

Side effects from taking kava kava are generally mild: stomach upset and allergic skin reactions. Both clear up after supplementation is discontinued. Long-term use may cause yellow discoloration of the skin, allergic reactions, visual disturbances, inflammation of the eyes, and balance problems. That being so, Commission E recommends that kava kava be taken no longer than three months. If you want to stay on it for a longer period of time, you should be under medical supervision. Never exceed recommended dosages. Also, taking too much kava kava produces the same effects as alcohol intoxication. High doses may impair your ability to drive or to operate heavy equipment, and thus lead to serious, even fatal, accidents.

The German Commission E warns against using kava kava with alcohol, barbiturates, antidepressants, and other agents that act on the central nervous system.

Additionally, kava kava should not be taken if you are pregnant or nursing, or suffer from Parkinson's disease (kava kava may worsen the condition).

WHAT IS ST. JOHN'S WORT?

Unless you've been stranded on a desert island, you've no doubt heard of St. John's wort, a common herb grown throughout Europe and North America. Although it has been around for ages—the Greeks and Romans used it to treat infections and inflammation—St. John's wort has been much publicized in the media. Psychiatrist Harold H. Bloomfield's book *Hypericum and Depression* (Prelude Press) put the herb in the spotlight, where it has stayed ever since. And, in 1997, German and American researchers evaluated twenty-three studies of St. John's wort and concluded that it worked as well as, sometimes better than, prescription antidepressants for treating mild to moderate depression, a mental disorder that affects one out of four Americans. Best of all, the herbal treatment produced fewer side effects. In 1993, more than 2.7 million prescriptions were written in Germany for St. John's wort. In fact, it outsells Prozac seven to one. In the United States, the National Institutes of Health (NIH) has sunk $4.5 million into studying the effectiveness of St. John's wort.

HOW IT WORKS

The active compound in St. John's wort is hypericin, a chemical that was first isolated from the herb in 1942 and has a significant antidepressant effect. Some pharmacologists think other active ingredients besides hypericin may be at work. Benefits from supplementing with St. John's wort include the following:

· Relief of depression

· Elevation of mood

· Relief of anxiety

· Increased sense of well-being

· Enhanced sleep

· Alertness.

The herb is believed to increase serotonin levels in the brain, although no one knows exactly how. Elevated serotonin levels tend to suppress the appetite and curb carbohydrate cravings.

St. John's wort's effect on serotonin levels is one reason why it is an ingredient in certain natural weight-loss supplements. Sometimes it is combined with 5-HTP (see chapter 6), a building block of serotonin, presumably to enhance the effects of this brain chemical. However, no scientific evidence exists to support any benefit from a St. John's wort/5-HTP combo.

At least one product combines St. John's wort with the amino acid phenylalanine—a formulation that claims to help build neurotransmitters (both the herb and the amino acid increase levels of neurotransmitters in the brain). In theory, this combination should work, but again, there are no data available to support the effectiveness of such a formulation.

Some formulas pair St. John's wort with the herbal stimulant ephedra, which contains ephedrine, known to help the body burn fat. An active compound called catechin in St. John's wort apparently extends the half-life of ephedrine—in other words, it guards ephedrine so that it stays in the body longer before being eliminated. Theoretically, the longer ephedrine stays in the body, the more time it has to exert its fat-burning action. But this is all supposition. No studies, animal or human, are yet available. Besides, ephedra is a stimulant, and St. John's wort is an anti-depressant. This could produce a tug-of-war effect on the system, with adverse side effects and imbalances. (For more on this issue, see chapter 13.)

It's extremely important to read the labels of natural weight-loss supplements and educate yourself on the ingredients they contain, and what they can and cannot do. (A partial list of natural weight-loss supplements and their ingredients is featured in appendix C.)

HOW TO USE IT

St. John's wort seems best used temporarily to improve mood, and thus prevent depression-related overeating. The usual dosage is two capsules daily (200 mg to 300 mg) of a capsulized product standardized to 0.3 percent hypericin. Teas and tincture usually don't deliver reliable doses.

It takes about 2 to 4 weeks for the herb to take effect. Unlike many prescription anti-depressants, there are no withdrawal symptoms from discontinuing the use of St. John's wort. Nor is the herb addictive.

SAFETY CONSIDERATIONS

Some bad news here for dieters: Unfortunately, one of the side effects of St. John's wort is weight gain—which can be quite discouraging. If you're considering St. John's wort to battle emotional overeating, you must weigh the consequences: Can you endure a temporary weight gain while you get your emotions under control, or will the weight gain make you more apt to binge?

St. John's wort can also make your skin more sensitive to light. That means you'll be more likely to get a sunburn if you go outside. If you're fair-skinned and supplementing with St. John's wort, avoid sunlight.

St. John's wort has been used extensively in Germany with no published reports of serious side effects. Observations on 3,250 patients taking the supplement noted that the most common side effects were gastrointestinal symptoms (0.6 percent), allergic reactions (0.5 percent), and fatigue (0.4 percent).

The herb should not be taken in conjunction with other drugs that affect serotonin levels, such as fluoxetine (Prozac) and monoamine oxidase (MAO) inhibitors. If it is taken with these drugs, serious side effects could result, including high blood pressure and a dangerous condition called the serotonin syndrome. This syndrome is marked by sweating, agitation, upset stomach, and jerky muscles. Severe reactions cause seizures, coma, even death.

As with any supplement, do not take St. John's wort if you are pregnant or nursing, or suffer from any disease. Antidepressants such as St. John's wort should be taken under medical supervision. If you suffer from emotional or binge eating, seek counseling to discover the underlying reasons for your behavior.

BATTLING BINGES

Occasional splurges are nothing to fret over. But when splurges become habitual binges, you've got cause for alarm. Here are some suggestions for battling binges:

· Clear the kitchen cabinets of binge food if you're prone to episodes of emotional overeating.

· Purchase single servings of any food you're likely to binge on. That way, you're less likely to eat the whole bag, the whole carton, the whole anything.

· Fill up on high-fiber foods. They take up a lot of space in your stomach, so you're less likely to gorge on them.

· Exercise regularly to relieve anxiety and depression.

· Distract yourself with a nonfood-related activity, like exercising, reading, pursuing a favorite hobby, listening to music, writing letters, surfing the Internet (one of the best distractions yet), or soaking in a hot bath.

· Make a list of fifty things to do other than overeat. Keep your list handy.

· If driving home from work takes you by your favorite drive-thru, find another route.

· Do you overeat or oversnack in front of the television? If so, make it a rule in your house always to eat in the dining room or kitchen.

· If you're vulnerable to oversnacking the moment you walk in the door after work, revamp your daily diet so that you're less ravenous. Make sure to eat a healthy snack at midmorning and midafternoon, and don't skip lunch. Or instead of raiding the fridge after coming home, head to the gym.

THIRTEEN

HERBAL WEIGHT LOSS:
THE SKINNY ON FORTY-THREE DIET HERBS

Thousands of herbs are available worldwide for a dizzying array of diseases and disorders. And consumers are sold on them: A recent survey found that one in three people spends an average of $54 a year on herbal remedies.

Without question, herbs do work wonders in treating many illnesses and improving health. But herbal medicine has a far less effective track record when it comes to weight control. Only one herb—ephedra—is believed to directly promote fat-burning, but its dangerous side effects make it unsafe and unwise to use.

There is one particular aspect of your weight you can control to some extent by supplementing with herbs, and that is water weight. Let's say you weigh 150 pounds. About ninety of those pounds are water; thirty are fat. The rest is lean tissue—muscles, organs, and bones. So normally, most of your body weight is water. Sometimes you may retain water. You look and feel fat, even though you may have lost a significant amount of body fat. Some days, you can't even fit into clothes you wore the week before!

Puffiness does masquerade as pudge. Disheartening and uncomfortable, periodic bouts of water retention, medically known as edema, may be the result of any number of factors: excess sodium in the diet, food allergies, premenstrual changes, hormone imbalances, a hot climate, and kidney or heart disease. If you're chronically plagued by edema, have it checked out by your doctor.

You can lose some of that fluid by taking a prescription "water pill" (diuretic) or by forcing yourself to sweat in a sauna or steam bath. Neither is a good idea, though, because they can lead to life-threatening dehydration and mineral imbalances.

Some herbs, however, may offer a gentler solution. Most of the herbs promoted for weight loss are diuretics—agents that cause the kidneys to draw extra water from the blood into the urine and stimulate the excretion of water. This action promotes temporary water loss. There's certainly nothing wrong with regulating water weight by using herbs, as long as you use them on a short-term basis and with the full knowledge of your physician. In most cases, herbal diuretics are safer than their prescription counterparts. But long-term use of either can flush vital nutrients from the body and cause irreparable harm.

Other weight-loss herbs are really nothing more than laxatives, which also force water from the body. It's much healthier to follow a high-fiber diet and drink plenty of pure water daily than to rely on laxatives for elimination. Prolonged used of laxatives and diuretics, even natural ones, can lead to dependence and serious health problems.

What follows is a discussion of forty-three herbs commonly promoted as diet aids. In most cases, these herbs are found in natural weight-loss supplements in minute amounts, mainly as fillers. In others, they are single- or multiherb formulas, available as capsules, compressed tablets, liquids, extracts, or teas. It's a good practice to read the list of ingredients on any natural weight-loss supplement carefully. The information below will help you make informed decisions about specific products.

ALFALFA

What It Is

Alfalfa is a nourishing legume used worldwide to feed animals. Many people eat alfalfa sprouts on salads or in sandwiches. Nutritionally, alfalfa is rich in protein; vitamins A, B, D, and K; and several minerals, including iron and copper.

Fact and Fiction

As a food supplement, alfalfa is sold by health food stores in powder, tablet, juice, tea, and other forms. In a few studies, alfalfa has been shown to reduce levels of LDL cholesterol in the body. Reportedly, it has natural diuretic and laxative properties—which is why it shows up in some natural weight-loss supplements. No credible scientific evidence, however, supports any weight-loss benefits. Paradoxically, it has a reputation in folk medicine as an appetite stimulant.

Safety Considerations

Alfalfa is generally regarded as safe when used in the tiny amounts found in natural weight-loss supplements. Some herbalists, however, advise against using alfalfa or alfalfa products at all, since the sprouts and seeds have been found to be toxic when consumed in large quantities.

ALOE

What It Is

A member of the lily family, aloe is an African succulent plant. Its leaves are filled with an anti-bacterial and anti-fungal gel that appears to be useful as a topical agent for treating wounds and healing first-degree and second-degree burns, as well as X-ray or other radiation burns. The gel is also processed into juice and pills, taken internally for gastrointestinal problems. The rind yields a whitish substance that is a powerful laxative.

Fact and Fiction

Aloe shows up as a weight-loss herb because of its laxative effects. It contains powerful laxative chemicals known as anthraquinones. Most recently, aloe has been paired with hydroxyproline, a protein found in collagen, as part of a rather bogus liquid protein diet aid. (For more information on this product, see chapter 7.)

Safety Considerations

Aloe is so potent a laxative that credible authorities rarely recommend its use for treating constipation. Side effects may include abdominal cramping, bowel irritation, diarrhea, nausea, red urine, and vomiting.

ASTRAGALUS

What It Is

Astragalus comes from the root of a legume cultivated in Asia. It has been used for thousands of years in China as a restorative tonic.

Fact and Fiction

Various research studies have confirmed that astragalus has anti-bacterial, anti-viral, and anti-inflammatory properties. It is fast gaining an excellent reputation in natural medicine circles as an immune system booster. At least one natural weight-loss product on the market lists astragalus in its formulation, along with other ingredients. But despite its many true talents, astragalus has no effect on weight loss.

Safety Considerations

Astragalus is considered to be a safe herb. No toxic reactions have been reported in animals or humans even when the herb is taken in very large doses.

BLADDERWRACK

What It Is

Used in steam baths by Native Americans to treat joint problems and other illnesses, bladderwrack is a seaweed rich in iodine, a mineral required by the body in tiny amounts and an essential component of thyroid hormones. An iodine deficiency is usually related to hypothyroidism (an underactive thyroid). People with this condition are prone to weight gain.

Fact and Fiction

Because it is high in iodine, bladderwrack is thought to correct a sluggish thyroid, thus boosting the metabolism and treating obesity. Bladderwrack is a familiar homeopathic weight-loss herb in Europe and has been available in American health food stores for several years. Its benefit in promoting weight loss is purely speculative, however.

Safety Considerations

If you suspect you have a weight-related thyroid problem, see your physician before self-medicating with an herbal preparation. (For more information on the risks involved in iodine supplementation, see the section below on kelp.)

BUCHU

What It Is

Derived from a shrub native to South Africa, the leaves of this herb are usually made into a tea and other supplement forms.

Fact and Fiction

Buchu is a known diuretic and antiseptic that fights germs in the urinary tract.

Safety Considerations

It is generally considered safe, though herbalists recommend taking no more than 2 grams two or three times a day.

BUCKTHORN

What It Is

The bark of the thorny buckthorn shrub is used to make various herbal preparations, including tea. Its berries go into the manufacturing of dyes and syrups.

Fact and Fiction

Like aloe, this herb contains powerful laxative chemicals called anthraquinones—which is why herbalists sometimes recommend it for chronic constipation.

Safety Considerations

Buckthorn is not a gentle laxative! It can cause severe diarrhea, nausea, vomiting, dangerously low blood pressure, and kidney damage (with prolonged use).

A 1989 article published in *American Family Physician* related a case study in which an eighty-year-old woman, appearing disoriented and confused, was seen for a second time in the emergency room. Her symptoms included diarrhea and orthostatic hypotension—abnormally low blood pressure that leads to dizziness or fainting upon getting up from a seated position. After she was given fluids, the woman's condition improved. It turned out that she drank a lot of buckthorn tea—a habit her physician advised against. This herb is risky; there's no rational reason to use it therapeutically.

BURDOCK

What It Is

Burdock has been used since ancient times as a healing remedy. Today, its leaves and seeds are formulated into herbal preparations.

Fact and Fiction

Burdock contains chemicals considered to be anti-bacterial, anti-fungal, tumor-protective, and diuretic. None of these claims has been verified scientifically.

Safety Considerations

Burdock appears to be safe, although it may interfere with the absorption of iron and other minerals.

CAPSICUM (CAYENNE PEPPER, RED PEPPER)
What It Is

Capsicum is the red pepper with which you spice your foods. It contains a number of active chemicals and is available as a condiment, in powder form, and as a cream applied topically to relieve joint pain.

Fact and Fiction

Capsicum is added to natural weight-loss products because it is believed to stimulate the metabolism by creating heat. You've probably noticed this yourself. After you eat hot, spicy foods, your body heats up. When body heat rises, so does metabolism, and more calories are burned. At least one study has measured the metabolic rates of people who ate capsicum with meals. When a teaspoon of red-pepper sauce and a teaspoon of mustard were added to meals, metabolic rates rose by as much as 25 percent.

There is little other evidence to prove capsicum's effect on weight loss. But it has many other health benefits attributed to the pain-relieving chemicals it contains. One is capsaicin, which triggers the release of endorphins and is found in topical creams recommended to ease arthritis pain. Capsaicin also inhibits substance P, which is believed to help transmit pain signals to and from the brain. Capsicum also contains aspirin-like chemicals called salicylates.

Safety Considerations

Capsicum is safe when used in very small amounts to spice foods, as a filler in supplements, or as a topical ointment to relieve joint pain.

CASCARA SAGRADA
What It Is

Cascara sagrada is a stimulant found in some natural weight-loss supplements and over-the-counter laxatives.

Fact and Fiction

It forces water from the body, creating the illusion of weight loss. Watery, explosive diarrhea is often the result.

Safety Considerations

Long-term use could cause dependence and heart problems, due to depletion of electrolytes from the body. Electrolytes are minerals that help control vital functions such as heart rhythm. Cascara sagrada is considered slightly dangerous and should be used with extreme caution, if at all.

CHICKWEED

What It Is

Chickweed is an herb high in vitamin C, and various parts of the plant are used in herbal preparations.

Fact and Fiction

Chickweed gets its reputation as a slimming agent from folk medicine; there is no scientific evidence to support this claim. The herb has diuretic properties, however, and may produce a temporary loss of water weight.

Safety Considerations

Chickweed is considered to be relatively safe when taken in recommended doses for short periods of time.

CINNAMON

What It Is

Cinnamon, derived from a tree of the laurel family, is everyone's favorite spice.

Fact and Fiction

In addition to spicing foods, cinnamon is used as a medicine—to treat nausea, relieve stomach gas, and reduce fevers. In one scientific experiment, the spice was found to help the body better digest sweets by improving the ability of insulin to move sugar into cells. It has been described as an herbal lipotropic (an agent that removes fat from storage or prevents its buildup in the body). A few natural weight-loss supplements contain traces of cinnamon; however, it has no proven effect on fat loss.

Safety Considerations

Cinnamon is very safe.

CITRUS AURANTIUM (BITTER ORANGE, SYNEPHRINE)

What It Is

Citrus aurantium is the botanical name of the Chinese fruit zhishi. An alkaloid called synephrine is extracted from this fruit and used as an ingredient in several natural weight-loss supplements. Both synephrine and its source, citrus aurantium, are found in marmalade.

Synephrine is a chemical cousin of ephedrine (an alkaloid found in the herb ephedra) but has few of ephedrine's adverse side effects. This is because synephrine, unlike ephedrine, does not easily cross the blood-brain barrier, and therefore cannot stimulate the central nervous system. (See the section below on ephedra.)

Fact and Fiction

Synephrine is thought to suppress the appetite, increase the metabolic rate, and help burn fat. Scientists believe that it works by activating cellular receptors—structures mounted on the surfaces of fat cells. When certain types of receptors are activated, the action of fat-burning enzymes inside the fat cell increases and fat is burned. Ephedrine is believed to stimulate fat cells in much that manner. Additionally, preliminary research on synephrine hints that it may do a better job than ephedrine at raising the metabolic rate. In fact, studies have shown that supplementing with synephrine burns as many as 128 extra calories a day, or nearly 900 calories a week—so far, without any negative side effects on the heart or blood pressure.

EAS, a supplement manufacturer, conducted a preliminary test on one of its natural weight-loss supplements, a product called Phen-Free. It is formulated with synephrine, caffeine, cordyceps (see p. 134), and other nutrients. Seven healthy men and women were recruited for the study—four were weight-trainers, and three were nonexercisers. Using a sophisticated test, the researchers first assessed the volunteers' metabolic rate, body temperature, and fuel utilization (a measure of how much fat or carbohydrate is burned). One week later, the same assessment was applied, with one exception. The volunteers took a dose (four capsules) of Phen-Free half an hour prior to the assessment. Remarkably, supplementation with Phen-Free boosted fat-burning by more than 18 percent.

If synephrine turns out to be as good as it sounds, it could be a powerful natural fat-burner. But to date, not enough is known about its exact effects.

Safety Considerations

Proceed with caution until more is known about the safety of citrus aurantium and its active component, synephrine. Even manufacturers who formulate supplements containing citrus aurantium are issuing caveats. Case in point: A product called Synephrinol, which contains pure citrus aurantium along with some caffeine-containing herbs, carries the following contraindications on its label: "Do not consume this product if you have high blood pressure, prostatic hypertrophy [enlarged prostate], hyperthyroidism, glaucoma, cardiac arrhythmias, or pheochromocytoma [an adrenal gland tumor that causes overproduction of epinedrine or norepinephrine]. This product should not be consumed in combination with MAO (monoamine oxidase) inhibitors or with any antidepressant drug which blocks the transport of norepinephrine. Curtail or discontinue use if nervousness, sleeplessness, or nausea occurs. Not intended for use by persons under the age of 18."

CORDYCEPS

What It Is

Cordyceps is a mushroom native to mountainous regions of China and Tibet. It is unusual in that it grows on caterpillar larvae.

Fact and Fiction

This mushroom has been used for centuries in China as a food and as a tonic to boost immunity, alleviate fatigue, fight old age, and strengthen the lungs, kidneys, and reproductive system. It is more of a folk remedy than a proven medicine.

Cordyceps is available as a supplement and is found as an ingredient in some natural weight-loss supplements. However, no one knows if cordyceps has any direct effect on weight loss.

Most likely, the reason cordyceps is included in multinutrient weight-loss products is its possible effect on exercise performance. In fact, many Chinese athletes swear by cordyceps. Some researchers think that it opens up breathing passages to let more oxygen circulate. With more oxygen available to cells, endurance increases.

Safety Considerations

Cordyceps is described as safe and gentle, but very little information exists on its safety. Some people in China use it once a week; others, daily.

CORNSILK

What It Is

The long, fibrous filaments on an ear of corn are cornsilk. As an herbal preparation, it is dried into powder and placed in capsules.

Fact and Fiction

Cornsilk does not affect fat loss but is a natural diuretic to help rid the body of excess water. The Chinese use it to reduce swelling (edema) caused by kidney disease. In one study of twelve kidney patients taking 2 ounces of cornsilk twice a day, edema completely disappeared in nine of the subjects.

Safety Considerations

Cornsilk is a harmless herb.

CRANBERRY

What It Is

Cranberry supplements are made from the familiar red berries of an evergreen native to North America. The juice of the berries is dried into a powder or concentrated as an extract, and put into capsules or tablets.

Fact and Fiction

This powder is a filler in some natural weight-loss supplements, probably because cranberry is somewhat diuretic and able to prevent water retention. The diuretic component of cranberry is a natural chemical called arbutin. Arbutin is also an antibiotic and the active ingredient that fights urinary tract infections.

Safety Considerations

Cranberry is considered very safe.

DANDELION

What It Is

Dandelion—the stubborn weed that pops up in your lawn every spring—is actually a healthful herb packed with vitamin A, vitamin C, and various minerals, particularly potassium.

Fact and Fiction

Its ground roots and leaves are used in herbal medicine for a variety of ailments, including water retention. Studies have confirmed its power as a diuretic—a safe one, too, since the herb's high potassium content replaces any potassium lost in the urine. Also, dandelion is thought to be an herbal lipotropic, although no evidence exists to support this claim.

Safety Considerations

Dandelion is considered very safe.

EPHEDRA

What It Is

Ephedra is a plant that contains ephedrine alkaloids, stimulant compounds that act on the appetite control center of the brain to suppress appetite. Ephedrine also stimulates the heart and central nervous system much as amphetamines do. Dietary supplements containing ephedrine are sold as weight-loss agents, energy boosters, and bodybuilding aids. Cold remedies also contain ephedrine. Ephedra goes by other names as well: ma huang, Mormon tea, Brigham tea, and popotillo.

Fact and Fiction

Chemically, ephedrine resembles our body's own stimulant, adrenaline (epinephrine), which, among other functions, liberates fat from cells to be used as energy. That is why you find the herb ephedra in many weight-loss supplements.

Accompanying ephedra in many of these formulations are caffeine-containing agents, such as guarana, green tea, and yerba maté. Like ephedrine, caffeine is believed to stimulate the production of fat-releasing adrenaline. And when combined with ephedra, caffeine reportedly doubles thermogenesis (the creation of body heat). Studies in Denmark showed that a drug made of ephedrine and caffeine was helpful in promoting weight loss; however, the combination produced central nervous system side effects such as agitation.

Ephedrine and caffeine were tested against dexfenfluramine (Redux), which has been removed from the market. In the most overweight people, the ephedrine/caffeine combo was found to be 29 percent more effective for weight loss than dexfenfluramine.

To burn fat, some bodybuilders and exercisers use something called a caffeine/ephedrine/aspirin stack. This is a combination of, usually, 20 mg of ephedrine, 200 mg of caffeine, and 300 mg of aspirin. Including aspirin supposedly regulates body temperature to preserve the thermogenic effect. This combination also seems to reduce appetite.

A 1993 study looked into the effectiveness of the caffeine/ephedrine/ aspirin combo on weight loss. Over an 8-week period, people taking the combination lost nearly 12 pounds—without exercising or cutting calories. Those given a placebo didn't do as well.

The caffeine/ephedrine/aspirin stack may be risky, however, since ephedrine has so many troublesome side effects (see below). Caffeine may aggravate certain health problems, such as ulcers, heart disease, high blood pressure, and anemia, to name just a few. Aspirin can upset your stomach.

Safety Considerations

Ephedrine often produces adverse reactions, including sleeplessness, anxiety, and nervousness. It can make the heart race and blood pressure soar. Because of these effects, people with heart conditions, high blood pressure, or diabetes should stay away from it.

When abused, ephedra and ephedrine can be lethal. In 1993, neurologists from the University of New Mexico reported that ephedrine had caused strokes in three people who had exceeded the recommended dosages.

In June 1997, in an attempt to curb the health problems associated with ephedra and supplements containing it, the FDA proposed safety measures that would result in marketing and label changes. The proposal would forbid the marketing of dietary supplements containing 8 mg or more of ephedrine alkaloids per serving. Also, a total daily intake of 24 mg or more would not be allowed. Labels would instruct consumers to not take the product for more than seven days. A warning would appear on labels, too: "Taking more than the recommended serving may result in heart attack, stroke, seizure, or death."

Also proposed was a ban on formulating products containing ephedrine plus other stimulant products such as herbal sources of caffeine. Such combinations increase the stimulant effects of ephedrine and the chance of serious side effects. (Manufacturers of over-the-counter cold and flu medications that contain ephedrine and the less potent pseudoephedrine would not be affected by these regulations.)

Since 1994, the FDA has received and investigated more than 800 complaints of health problems associated with the use of ephedrine-containing products. Among the most serious: heart attacks, stroke, and death. Most occurred in young-to-middle-aged, otherwise healthy adults using the products for weight control and increased energy. Clearly, the risks of supplementing with ephedra products outweigh any benefits.

FENNEL

What It Is

Fennel is a member of the same plant family as carrots and parsley. Its seeds, roots, and stems are made into herbal preparations.

Fact and Fiction

Herbalists recommend fennel for treating a variety of ailments, including asthma, upset stomach, angina, and breast-feeding problems. You may find it listed on the labels of a few natural weight-loss supplements, but it has no effect on fat loss.

Safety Considerations

Fennel is a trace ingredient in natural diet products and is considered to be safe.

FLAX

What It Is

Flax contains important essential fats and has been attracting attention for its many disease-fighting benefits. It is available as an oil, flour, whole seeds, or pulverized in supplements.

Fact and Fiction

Several years ago at the annual Convention on Experimental Biology, the Food and Drug Administration (FDA) and several other research institutions presented evidence that flax does the following:

- Helps stimulate the immune system

- Increases the retention of vitamin D and several minerals

- Has anti-tumor properties

- Is high in antioxidants

- Lowers triglyceride levels and favorably alters cholesterol profiles.

But despite these remarkable attributes, flax has no effect on fat loss. The reason it shows up in natural weight-loss supplements is that it works as a natural laxative, forming bulk in the intestinal tract and thus aiding in elimination.

Safety Considerations

In its various forms, flax is very safe and healthy.

GINGER ROOT

What It Is

Used since ancient times, this herb is processed from the underground stem of a tropical plant native to Asia. It is available in tablets, capsules, tea, extracts, and syrups, and as a filler in a few natural weight-loss supplements.

Fact and Fiction

Ginger root, which contains a number of beneficial chemicals, has a long list of bona fide medical uses: relieving intestinal gas, treating nausea caused by motion sickness, and reducing joint inflammation, to name just a few. This versatile, healthful herb, however, has no effect on fat loss.

Safety Considerations

Supplementing with ginger root is very safe.

GINSENG

What It Is

There are three types of ginseng: the Asian variety (*Panax ginseng*); American ginseng (*Panax quinquefolius*); and Siberian ginseng (*Eleutherococcus senticosus*), a different species than *Panax*. Siberian ginseng is not a true ginseng, but a botanical cousin. It is the same plant as the Chinese herb known as ciwujia. (See chapter 14.)

Fact and Fiction

Derived from the roots and leaves of a thorny shrub, Siberian ginseng has been studied extensively. Research shows that it may increase energy, extend endurance, ward off fatigue, and enhance the immune system. In Russia, it has been used by cosmonauts and Olympic athletes to boost

energy and fight the effects of stress. The herb's active ingredients, called
eleutherosides, are thought to be responsible for Siberian ginseng's many
health benefits.

Derived from the plant's root, the Asian and American forms of
ginseng are the two varieties most commonly used in the West. Their active
particles, termed ginsenocides, have benefits similar to those of eleutherosides. Some research shows that ginsenosides may halt the buildup of
plaque in the arteries and reduce cancer risk by preventing cell damage
caused by free radicals. Nearly 2,900 scientific studies have been conducted
on ginseng, mainly the Asian variety.

Ginseng has a reputation as an aphrodisiac, an adaptogen (a stress-
resisting agent), an anabolic (tissue-builder), and an antioxidant. There's
no proof that ginseng enhances sexual performance or potency. But there's
some evidence that it may positively influence stress. Animal studies show
some tissue-building reaction to ginseng taken orally; however, researchers
haven't been able to replicate those results in humans.

From a weight-loss perspective, ginseng supposedly can treat water
retention. But proof of this benefit is sketchy. Ginseng is also among a
handful of herbs reputed to be lipotropic.

Of interest to exercisers and athletes is ginseng's possible effect on
physical performance. Italian researchers investigated the stamina-producing
powers of ginseng. They studied fifty male sports teachers, all healthy, ages
21 to 47 years. Every 6 weeks, the participants took two capsules
containing either ginseng extract, vitamins, and minerals, or placebos.
After taking either the ginseng preparation or the placebo, they exercised
on a treadmill at increasing workloads. The ginseng group performed
much better than the placebo subjects. This finding led the researchers to
conclude that the ginseng preparation boosted performance by improving
the supply of oxygen to the muscles.

In China today, many preparations of ginseng are officially approved
for medicinal use. You find ginseng in teas and as powders, capsules,
extracts, tablets, and ginseng-flavored soft drinks.

Safety Considerations

Authorities generally regard ginseng as safe if taken in minimal
quantities for short periods of time. There are known side effects of large
doses and long-term use: diarrhea, insomnia, nervousness, nausea, and
vomiting.

GOTU KOLA

What It Is

A member of the parsley family, gotu kola is a common weed that grows in drainage ditches in Asia and orchards in Hawaii.

Fact and Fiction

Folk tradition says that if you eat a leaf of gotu kola every day, you'll live to be 1,000! It's reputed to be an anti-aging herb, an aphrodisiac, a memory restorative, and a wound healer. As you might guess, there's no evidence to support these claims. A known effect of this herb is that it fights water retention by helping the body eliminate excess fluid. It is also a central nervous system stimulant and is believed to be a lipotropic herb.

Safety Considerations

Gotu kola is relatively safe if taken on a short-term basis. However, it should be avoided if you have a chronic medical condition because of its stimulating effect. Side effects include insomnia and nervousness.

GREEN TEA EXTRACT

What It Is

Green tea comes from the leaves and leaf buds of an evergreen tree native to Asia. An extract standardized for a beneficial group of chemicals called polyphenols is made from the tea and put into capsules or used as a filler in some natural weight-loss supplements.

Fact and Fiction

Green tea and its extract have a number of beneficial properties. Research shows that they may protect against certain cancers, enhance cardiovascular health, and boost fat metabolism (which is one reason you find it in natural weight-loss supplements). Green tea contains some caffeine, but less than half of what you get in coffee. Caffeine is believed to help release fatty acids into the bloodstream for use as energy.

Safety Considerations

Unless you're sensitive to caffeine, green tea or extracts containing it are very safe and probably beneficial to health.

GUARANA

What It Is

Guarana is a red berry from a plant grown in the Amazon valley. It contains seven times as much caffeine as the coffee bean and is widely sold in health food stores as a supplement to increase energy. The supplement is made from the seeds of the berry.

Fact and Fiction

Guarana is used in a number of natural weight-loss supplements, often combined with ephedra. The combination is believed to increase thermogenesis (body heat), and thus to stimulate the metabolism. Guarana may also cause your body to lose water, since the caffeine it contains is a diuretic.

Safety Considerations

It is unwise to use guarana, especially with ephedra, because of its stimulating effects. Also, very high doses may disturb the heart and even cause panic attacks.

GYMNEMA SILVESTRE

What It Is

Gymnema silvestre is an herb derived from the leaves of a tree native to Africa and India. It is a member of the botanical family Asclepiadacerae, named after the Greek god of healing, Asclepius. The herb may reduce your desire for sugar by blocking the taste for sweets. In fact, the Hindu name for this herb is gurmar, which means "sugar killer."

Fact and Fiction

Gymnema has long been used in India to help treat diabetes, and many modern studies show that it can increase the production and activity of insulin, reduce blood sugar levels, and lower levels of blood fats. The active ingredient in gymnema, gymnemic acid, has been shown to block sugar absorption in the body.

As for weight loss, gymnema may be of some benefit if you have a sweet tooth and need to cut your consumption of sugary treats. (This benefit is largely untested, however. Even so, gymnema may be worth a try if you crave sweets.) Herbalists recommend taking gymnema extract before a large meal to reduce the appetite as well as quell cravings for sweets. Gymnema also has a reputation as a diuretic.

Safety Considerations

Gymnema is safe, and herbalists advise taking 150 mg of the extract three times a day. If you're a diabetic, do not supplement with gymnema without checking with your physician, since the herb affects sugar metabolism.

HAWTHORN

What It Is

Hawthorn preparations are made from the flowers, leaves, or berries of a thorny plant grown in Europe. In Germany and other parts of Europe, hawthorn extracts are widely prescribed to treat heart problems, high blood pressure, and arthritis. The herb is usually sold in capsule form, and infrequently is used as a filler in natural weight-loss supplements.

Fact and Fiction

Studies show that the herb dilates coronary arteries, thus improving blood flow and oxygen supply to the heart. But medical experts warn that hawthorn should be used only under a doctor's care. Even though you occasionally find it in tiny amounts in natural weight-loss products, there's no evidence that the herb has any benefit in weight control.

Safety Considerations

Hawthorn is a potent herb that should be used only under a doctor's supervision. However, so little hawthorn is used in natural weight-loss supplements that you shouldn't have to worry about taking it in such minute doses.

HORSETAIL

What It Is

A close relative of a tree that grew in dinosaur days, this herb is a rich source of silicon, a trace mineral involved in tissue repair. Among the chemicals it contains is nicotine.

Fact and Fiction

Herbalists have recommended horsetail to treat a wide range of conditions, including osteoporosis, bronchitis, balding, kidney problems, and bladder disorders. The research supporting its healing ability is scant, however. As for weight loss, horsetail is supposedly a diuretic, but this has not been proved conclusively.

Safety Considerations

Medical authorities rate horsetail as slightly dangerous. It is found in a few natural diet products, but only in small, benign amounts.

JUNIPER BERRY

What It Is

If you've ever sipped a dry martini, the flavor of the gin in your cocktail comes from the juniper berry.

Fact and Fiction

Because it reportedly contains a potent anti-viral compound, herbalists sometimes recommend juniper for fighting viruses, including those of the cold, flu, and herpes. Juniper is also billed as a diuretic, but this effect has not been documented medically.

Safety Considerations

This herb is considered to be slightly dangerous, since it is known to irritate the kidneys and interfere with the absorption of iron and other minerals. If included as part of a natural diet product, juniper berry is found in benign, trace amounts.

KELP

What It Is

During weight loss, thyroid hormone levels can drop—one reason why metabolism—and consequently fat-burning—often slows to a crawl while you're dieting. To pick up the pace, some nutritionists suggest supplementing with kelp, a nutritious sea vegetable loaded with iodine. Iodine is a trace mineral that helps the thyroid gland produce thyroxin, the principal thyroid hormone involved in metabolism. Tablets made from dehydrated kelp are often packaged as part of a weight-loss program that includes vinegar and vitamin B_6 (which works as a diuretic).

Fact and Fiction

There is no medical proof that kelp promotes weight loss, alone or in combination with vinegar and vitamin B_6. In 1991, the FDA banned kelp as an ingredient in over-the-counter diet drugs, because of unproved effectiveness. However, it is still sold in many natural diet aids as a weight-loss agent.

Safety Considerations

A potentially serious problem with kelp supplementation is over-consumption of iodine. The recommended daily allowance (RDA) for iodine is 150 micrograms—which you can easily obtain by drinking a cup of milk or salting your food with less than a half teaspoon of iodized salt. Many commercial baked goods contain iodine, too. At levels of more than 2,000 micrograms—an amount only a few times higher than the amount we get daily—iodine is quite toxic. It can cause an enlarged thyroid and disrupt the normal functioning of thyroid hormones. Iodine supplements, including kelp, should be avoided unless prescribed by your physician.

LICORICE

What It Is

You probably think of licorice as a black, chewy candy, but it is also an important herb used to treat inflammation and bronchial congestion. Licorice is derived from the roots and underground stem of a European plant and is available in capsules, powders, lozenges, and extracts. A few natural weight-loss supplements use it as an ingredient in tiny quantities.

Fact and Fiction

The active compound in licorice responsible for its therapeutic benefits is glycyrrhizin, which gives the herb its sweetness. Licorice also contains an anti-oxidant that may help prevent hardening of the arteries (technically known as atherosclerosis). There are no weight-loss benefits linked to licorice or to glycyrrhizin, however.

Safety Considerations

Supplementing with high or long-term doses of licorice extracts containing glycyrrhizin is dangerous because it may aggravate heart or kidney problems. Natural weight-loss supplements with licorice contain only traces of the extract, however. A modified form of licorice called DGL is considered safer.

MILK THISTLE

What It Is

Derived from a weedlike plant grown in the Mediterranean area, this herb has been used as liver protectant since ancient times.

Fact and Fiction

For more than 60 years, hundreds of studies have confirmed milk thistle's benefit on liver health. Most supplements contain standardized extracts of the herb's active ingredient, silymarin, and are used to treat cirrhosis, hepatitis, and other liver diseases, particularly in Europe. Where weight loss is concerned, milk thistle is thought to be an herbal lipotropic that helps remove fatty substances from the liver.

Safety Considerations

Supplementing with milk thistle and products containing it appears to be safe.

MUSTARD SEED

What It Is

The seed of the mustard plant is ground into a powder and often is found as an ingredient in natural weight-loss supplements. It is high in the mineral magnesium.

Fact and Fiction

Though it is a common ingredient in weight-loss products, mustard seed powder has no proven role in weight control.

Safety Considerations

Mustard seed powder is considered safe.

PARSLEY

What It Is

You know it best as a garnish on your dinner plate, but parsley has a reputation as a healer dating back to ancient times. And no wonder. It is very nutritious, rich in vitamin A, folic acid, iron, and other minerals.

Fact and Fiction

Therapeutically, parsley can decrease blood pressure and aid in digestion. It is a proven natural diuretic and thus may produce a slight loss of water weight.

Safety Considerations

Parsley is considered very safe.

PASSION FLOWER

What It Is

Passion flower is a perennial vine that grows in the eastern United States and is available as an herbal remedy.

Fact and Fiction

The herb exerts a sedative action, and has been found to relieve anxiety and reduce high blood pressure. At least one natural weight-loss supplement on the market lists passion flower as an ingredient, but there is no proof that it has any effect on weight loss. However, passion flower may help curb stress-related eating binges.

Safety Considerations

Passion flower appears to be safe, and the German Commission E has officially approved it for nervous anxiety.

PLANTAIN

What It Is

Plantain is a leafy plant approved by The German Commission E for treating sore throat, inflammation of the mucous membranes of the mouth and throat, and skin inflammation. The herb acts mainly as an astringent and an antibacterial.

Fact and Fiction

An Italian study has confirmed a weight-loss effect with plantain. Women who were severely obese (at least 60 percent over their recommended weight) supplemented with 3 grams of plantain in water half an hour prior to meals. The plantain-supplemented group lost more weight than a control group who simply cut calories. Supposedly, plantain reduces the absorption of fats and makes you feel full—which would explain its weight-loss benefit.

Safety Considerations

In 1977, the FDA issued a warning to consumers that they should stop using dietary supplements with plantain because the products may contain a toxic, digitalis-like substance. Digitalis is the active ingredient in some prescription heart medicines and a powerful heart stimulant. Digitalis can cause nausea, vomiting, dizziness, headache, low blood pressure, and abnormal heart rate and rhythm, including cardiac arrest.

Reportedly, the substance was detected in samples of raw material labeled as plantain and used in herbal laxatives and tea. The FDA swung into action after receiving a report of a life-threatening heart abnormality in a young woman who had supplemented with a product containing plantain. The news on plantain makes it potentially deadly and not to be fooled with if you're trying to lose weight.

SCHISANDRA

What It Is

This herb comes from the fruit of the schisandra shrub, cultivated in China.

Fact and Fiction

Schisandra is popular among herbalists as a liver protector. The herb is also used to treat colds, urinary incontinence, and allergies. It is unclear why schisandra is an ingredient in natural weight-loss supplements, since it has no effect on fat loss, nor is it a diuretic.

Safety Considerations

Schisandra is widely used in China, but very little information is available on its safety or effectiveness.

SENNA

What It Is

Senna is derived from the leaves of a shrub grown in India and is the active ingredient in several over-the-counter laxatives.

Fact and Fiction

Senna is a strong laxative. It stimulates contractions of the colon to relieve constipation.

Safety Considerations

Side effects include severe cramps, violent diarrhea, dehydration, and electrolyte imbalance. Some dieter's teas contain senna. It may produce a temporary loss of water weight, but it is neither effective nor safe if used as a weight-loss agent. Long-term use can lead to laxative dependence.

SPIRULINA

What It Is

Also known as blue-green algae, spirulina has been a popular supplement for years, thanks to its "superfood" reputation. Nutritionally, spirulina is a treasure trove of health-giving nutrients: beta carotene, B-vitamins, magnesium, and zinc.

Fact and Fiction

Spirulina has been touted as a curative for a range of conditions, including diabetes, liver disease, ulcers, and hair loss. But claims are largely without merit.

Spirulina has also been hailed as a weight-loss agent because it supposedly suppresses the appetite by increasing levels of the amino acid phenylalanine. In a Japanese study, diabetic patients were given twenty-one spirulina tablets a day, and within weeks, their symptoms improved, along with significant weight loss. Theoretically, the nutrient-packed spirulina reduced food cravings, which led to weight loss. However, more medical evidence is needed to verify whether spirulina affects appetite in any way.

Safety Considerations

There is really no harm in supplementing with spirulina. It's an expensive way to obtain nutrients you can get from food, however. Also, if grown in polluted water, spirulina may contain harmful microorganisms. High levels of mercury and other toxic metals have been detected in some batches.

UVA URSI

What It Is

This herb is derived from the leaves of the bearberry, an evergreen plant.

Fact and Fiction

A mild diuretic, uva ursi's active ingredients are ursolic acid and isoquercetin, two natural chemicals that increase urine output. Other compounds in uva ursi help prevent bacteria from anchoring to the uretha. Thus, the herb may be helpful in treating a mild urinary tract infection. But don't use it with cranberry juice or other acidic juices. They cancel out uva ursi's anti-bacterial effect.

Safety Considerations

Although considered relatively safe, uva ursi tends to turn urine green. If you have a sensitive stomach, this herb can cause nausea and vomiting. The small amounts of uva ursi used in natural diet products are generally harmless, however.

YELLOW DOCK

What It Is

The leaves and roots of yellow dock are used in herbal preparations. As a food, it has been used in salads.

Fact and Fiction

This herb is a laxative known for its stimulating action on the gastrointestinal tract. It has been recommended for treating occasional constipation experienced by dieters after altering their eating habits. Still, that's no reason to supplement with yellow dock. Eating a high-fiber diet and drinking plenty of fluids will usually correct such temporary constipation.

Safety Considerations

Yellow dock is considered slightly dangerous. Side effects include diarrhea, nausea, vomiting, and skin eruptions.

YERBA MATÉ
What It Is

Yerba maté is a South American plant whose leaves are dried and made into tea or put into capsules. The herb contains vitamins A, B-complex, and C, and the minerals calcium, magnesium, and iron.

Fact and Fiction

Yerba maté is usually touted as a natural upper. And for good reason: It is a central nervous system stimulant. But the herb's invigorating or fatigue-reducing effect is due mostly to its 2 percent caffeine content.

Yerba maté is found in some natural weight-loss supplements because it is believed to help control appetite, although there is no concrete proof of this. What is known, however, is that the herb has a mild diuretic effect. As with any diuretic, supplementing with it might produce temporary water weight loss.

Safety Considerations

Potential side effects of yerba maté may include confusion, excessive urination, irritability, nausea, nervousness, and rapid heartbeat. Consumed in very large amounts, yerba maté tea (also known as Paraguay tea) may be cancer-causing. (See the box on p. 155 on dieters' teas.) However, medical experts say the herb is relatively safe when taken in small quantities for short periods of time.

YOHIMBE
What It Is

Yohimbe is an herb derived from the bark of an evergreen grown in West Africa. It is best known for its aphrodisiac properties because it stimulates erection. An extract of the herb, yohimbine, is available as a prescription drug for treating erection problems.

Fact and Fiction

Yohimbine is an FDA-approved treatment for erection impairment, and it produces good results. What is less certain about the herb or its extract is its effect on fat loss. Yohimbine stimulates the release of noradrenaline (norepinephrine), a hormone that raises body temperature and helps liberate fatty acids from cells to be burned as fuel. When patients on a 1,000-calorie-a-day diet supplemented with yohimbine hydrochloride (a prescription medicine), they lost an average of 7.8 pounds in 3 weeks, compared with a control group who lost an average of 4.8 pounds. Whether or not the whole herb yohimbe produces the same effect is unclear. Still, the herb is included in some natural weight-loss formulas.

Safety Considerations

Yohimbe is considered a dangerous herb, even by herbalists' standards. It can cause anxiety, elevated blood pressure, irregular heartbeat, head-aches, painful erections, flushing, hallucinations, kidney failure, seizures, and death. The prescription form of the herb produces fewer side effects. This is one of those rare exceptions in which the raw herb is more toxic than its pharmaceutical cousin. It's best to avoid any natural weight-loss formula containing yohimbe. In fact, the American Botanical Council, which promotes herbal supplements, has recommended that consumers avoid it. Further, the FDA considers it to be potentially unsafe.

YUCCA

What It Is

The yucca plant is a member of the lily family that has been used by Native Americans in the southwestern United States to treat colds, flu, indigestion, and constipation.

Fact and Fiction

A 1992 article published in *Health News & Reviews* related the story of an anthropology professor who went on a diet of desert herbs, including yucca blossoms, and lost 30 pounds in 3 months. The truth be told, there is no scientific evidence supporting yucca as a weight-loss agent, although you may find it listed as an ingredient in some natural weight-loss products.

Safety Considerations

Yucca is probably safe in the trace amounts found in natural weight-loss supplements.

HERBAL PHEN-FEN PRODUCTS

In the wake of the ban against phen-fen and Redux, many weight-loss clinics began recommending "natural phen-fen" or "herbal phen-fen." Available at health food stores, these products are being hyped as safer, more natural alternatives to the now-banned diet drugs. However, herbal phen-fen may not be without risks.

The key ingredient in these formulas is ephedra, a powerful, nonprescription herbal stimulant that has been marketed heavily for weight loss. However, ephedra is linked to heart attacks, strokes, seizures, brain hemorrhages, and deaths. The FDA is keeping a close eye on ephedra. (See the section on ephedra.)

The other ingredient in herbal phen-fen is St. John's wort, an herb that depresses the central nervous system. According to a number of clinical trials, St. John's wort shows great promise in relieving mild depression and anxiety. But its side effects include weight gain, mild nausea, stomachache, tiredness, and sensitivity to sunlight. There is no evidence that St. John's wort leads to weight loss, although it might be helpful in reducing depression and thus fending off depression-related food binges. (See chapter 12 for more information on using St. John's wort in a weight-loss program.)

These herbs have opposing actions: Ephedrine is a stimulant, and St. John's wort is a depressant. No one really knows how such a combination could affect the body. Until more testing is done, there is no good rationale for supplementing with herbal phen-fen.

The FDA has herbal phen-fen producers on alert. In a position paper issued November 6, 1997, and posted on its Internet web site, the FDA said that it "considers these products to be unapproved drugs because their names reflect that they are intended for the same use as the anti-obesity drugs, fenfluramine and phentermine . . . FDA regards any over-the-counter product commercially promoted as an alternative to prescription anti-obesity drugs (such as phen-termine and fenfluramine) to be a drug. The agency is taking appropriate regulatory action to remove such products from the market."

In other words, companies selling herbal phen-fen supplements and labeling them as such have to be careful about how they promote, market, and name their natural diet aids. As soon as an ad, or even a product name, starts making the supplement sound like a drug, that is, that it can cure obesity, the product and its manufacturer may be in regulatory hot water. By law, supplements cannot expressly or implicitly claim to diagnose, treat, prevent, or cure a disease. If they do, they must be regarded as drugs and then must meet the safety and effectiveness standards for drugs.

SHOULD YOU DRINK DIETERS' TEAS?

Dieters' teas are among the herbal products in health food stores touted for weight loss—promoted by the words like "slim," "fat buster," "trim," "dieters'," or "calorie-free" on the packaging. Many of these teas contain laxatives such as aloe, senna, buckthorn, and cascara sagrada, which induce water loss and stimulate bowel movements.

Additionally, dieters' teas contain herbs that have a diuretic effect, also producing temporary weight reduction due to fluid loss.

Long-term use of these herbal teas can permanently impair the colon so that it may have to be surgically removed. Also, there have been several cases of heartbeat abnormalities and paralysis, and four deaths linked to these products. The deaths were probably a result of excessive loss of potassium from the body through diarrhea. Potassium is an important mineral, vital to the healthy functioning of the heart.

Some dieters' teas may also contain stimulants such as ma huang (ephedra) or yerba maté. As previously noted, ephedra can produce many unwanted side effects, including elevated blood pressure and heartbeat abnormalities. Yerba maté tea happens to be a popular beverage enjoyed in Uruguay. A study published in 1991 in the journal *Cancer* reported an alarming association between a high incidence of bladder cancer and maté tea-drinking among Uruguay natives. It's important to point out, however, that the natives drink up to two quarts a day of this tea, and the risk was particularly elevated if the tea drinkers also smoked black tobacco.

And in 1995, seven people in New York City suffered anticholinergic poisoning after drinking Paraquay tea, which is made from the yerba maté plant. The symptoms of this condition include agitation, flushed skin, fever, disorientation, and dilated pupils. Investigation and analysis by the New York City Department of Health, the New York City Poison Center, and the FDA concluded that the tea, shipped to New York grocery stores through a distributor who purchased it directly from South American farmers, had probably been contaminated with leaves from a plant containing active chemicals found in belladonna. Belladonna is a poisonous plant. In fact, there were nearly 1,000 reports in 1993 of poisonings caused by herbs contaminated with belladonna.

Does this mean you should forgo herbal teas altogether? Not at all. Herbal teas are a healthy alternative to caffeine-containing beverages. Teas with mint, rose hips, blackberry, raspberry, and chamomile, as well as those formulated with cold-fighting herbs like echinacea and goldenseal, and many others, are excellent beverages. However, if you should ever have an adverse reaction after taking any herbal preparation, see your physician right away.

SAFE WAYS TO BATTLE BLOAT

In cases where medical causes of fluid retention have been ruled out, here are three natural ways to help prevent bloat without resorting to any type of diuretic.

· Drink plenty of water throughout the day. Paradoxically, water is one of the best preventive measures against fluid retention. Your kidneys need a constant supply of water to properly eliminate fluids and waste products from your body. If water is in short supply, the kidneys tend to hoard water, and bloat can set in.

Additionally, drinking more water can actually help you stay lean, indirectly. Your kidneys rely on enough water to filter waste products from the body. In a water shortage, the kidneys need backup, so they turn to the liver for help. One of the liver's many functions is mobilizing stored fat for energy. By taking on extra assignments from the kidneys, the liver can't do its fat-burning job as well. Fat loss is compromised as a result. So try to drink between eight and ten glasses of pure water daily.

· Cut your sodium intake. Excessive salt also makes your body retain too much water. Salt your food lightly, and try to use less than half a teaspoon when fixing your meals. If you miss the taste of salt on your foods, try a salt substitute or experiment with various herbs and spices in your cooking.

· Maintain a regular aerobic exercise program. Aerobic exercise such as walking, jogging, or bicycling keeps blood vessels toned and resilient. If blood vessels lack resiliency, extra water can flow from them and collect in the tissues, causing water retention.

PART V

NATURAL WEIGHT CONTROL AND BEYOND

FOURTEEN

MORE DIET PRODUCTS: WHAT TO TRY, WHAT TO LEAVE ALONE

In addition to the weight-loss supplements already covered, there are several others on the market claiming to burn fat, accelerate metabolism, increase endurance, and confer a host of other benefits. Some look promising, but we just don't know enough about them yet. Others are downright dangerous or patently bogus. What follows is a look at these products—those worth a try and those better left alone.

WORTH A TRY

Conjugated Linoleic Acid (CLA)

What It Is: Discovered in 1978 at the University of Wisconsin, conjugated linoleic acid (CLA) is a naturally occurring fatty acid present in meat, dairy products (particularly cheddar and colby cheeses), sunflower oil, and safflower oil. It is formed when the bacteria in a cow's gut break down linoleic acid in the corn or soybeans the animal eats.

In 1996, CLA became available as a diet product derived from sunflower oil. Ads for CLA note that the nutrient may be missing from many diets (presumably since we tend to eat less meat and fewer high-fat dairy products). The product is promoted as a fat-burning, muscle-toning, energy-boosting agent and is included as a primary ingredient in many weight-loss supplements now on health food store shelves. Chromium picolinate is combined with CLA in some products.

How It Works: First of all, no one yet knows how, or if, CLA really exerts a fat-burning effect. Researchers think that the substance may interact with cytokines, nonantibody proteins that are involved in energy production and fat metabolism. They theorize that CLA somehow causes protein, carbohydrates, and fats to be used by cells for energy and muscle tissue growth, rather than to be stored as fat.

Cytokines are also involved in immunity. During an injury or illness, they signal the body to break down nonessential proteins (such as those in the skin) into amino acids, in order to manufacture antibodies and produce energy to fight the disease or injury.

In rat experiments, animals lost half their body fat and gained muscle tissue when fed the equivalent of 1 to 6 grams of CLA daily. In a human study involving CLA, twenty nonobese people (ten men and ten women) were given just over a gram of CLA or a placebo with breakfast, lunch, and dinner. They were instructed not to change their diet or exercise habits.

At the end of 3 months, the researchers measured both the weight and the body fat percentage of the study participants. Even though there was not much difference in weight loss between supplementers and nonsupplementers, there was a huge difference in body fat percentage. The CLA supplementers dropped from 21.3 percent (average body fat) to an average of 17 percent. While it might not sound like much, a reduction of a few points in body fat percentage can make a huge difference in how lean and firm you look. The people taking CLA lost mostly body fat—the ideal situation in any trim-down program.

Another study produced much different results. It looked into whether CLA would improve body composition (percentage of fat and muscle) and boost strength. But after twenty-eight days of supplementation and weight-training, CLA had no effect on either.

Other Benefits of CLA: While investigating carcinogens that occur in grilled meats, the researchers at the University of Wisconsin who first discovered CLA found that the fatty acid appeared to block the formation of cancer-causing substances rather than promoting them. This amazing finding led to more than a decade of intensive research on CLA's potential as a cancer-fighter. Many animal studies have since found that it suppresses mammary cancer and skin cancer.

A large-scale study conducted by Finland's National Public Health Institute, published in 1996, produced compelling evidence of CLA's anti-cancer benefit. Women who drank milk regularly for 25 years slashed their odds of getting breast cancer by 50 percent, compared with nonmilk-drinking women. The investigators zeroed in on CLA as the likely agent for the protective effect, since the fatty acid is highly concentrated in milk fat.

Animal research shows that CLA may also help prevent a wasting disease called cachexia, which occurs when the body burns up muscle to obtain energy for fighting diseases such as cancer. Cachexia compromises the survival of cancer patients. CLA has been shown to reverse muscle-wasting effects in diseased animals.

CLA is also considered to be an antioxidant. Animal studies have found that it may help clear the body of oxidized LDL cholesterol, a harmful substance that clogs arteries. Thus, CLA may help protect against heart disease, but further studies are needed to confirm this benefit.

How to Use It: Studies of CLA support a dosage of 2.5 to 5 grams a day if you are trying to lose body fat. Follow the manufacturer's recommendations for dosage.

Safety Considerations: Even though CLA shows tremendous promise, not enough is known about it to make a full judgment on its effectiveness. Still, it is worth a try if you're on a weight-reduction program.

By eating a varied diet that includes meat and dairy products in moderation, you should get adequate amounts of this nutrient. Gobbling hunks of cheese or swilling gallons of whole milk is not a good way to obtain CLA, since high-fat foods eaten in excess contribute to heart disease and other serious illnesses.

Ciwujia

What It Is: Pronounced su-wah-ja, ciwujia is extract of the root of a plant *(Acanthopanax senticosus)* grown in northeastern China. It is also known as Siberian ginseng.

In traditional Chinese medicine, ciwujia has been used for 1,700 years to prevent fatigue and boost immunity. The standardized extract of the root is available as a sports supplement; the best-known product is Endurox™ or Endurox® Excel™ (which contains vitamin E). Other ciwujia supplements on the market are formulated with ginseng, bee pollen, carbohydrates, and licorice.

Endurox® is promoted as a dietary aid to boost endurance, delay lactic acid buildup in muscles, and spare carbohydrates in favor of fat to fuel exercise. According to a survey released by the magazine *Inside Triathlon*, Endurox® is the nutritional supplement third most frequently used by triathletes. It is also endorsed by many professional athletes, including NFL superstar Joe Montana.

How It Works: Ciwujia stepped to nutritional center stage when it was learned that mountain climbers were using it to improve endurance and oxygen use at high altitudes. Interest in the herb grew.

Two studies of Endurox™ conducted at the Institute of Nutrition and Food Hygiene in Beijing, China, suggest that the herb increases fat-burning during exercise, in two ways. First, it shifts the body's fuel source from carbohydrates to fat. This means your body starts burning fat earlier in your workout. Second, supplementation retards the accumulation of lactic acid (this buildup accounts for the sensation in your muscles known as the "burn"). With less lactic acid, you can work out longer and harder—and burn more fat in the process.

In the first study, eight men were given 800 mg of Endurox® daily for 2 weeks prior to starting the experiment. By the end of 2 weeks, the men pedaled on stationary bikes with increasing levels of intensity. As the intensity went up, lactic acid levels in their muscles went down—by 33 percent. That's the opposite of what usually occurs when you work out. As exercise becomes harder, more and more lactic acid swells your muscles, and you discontinue the exercise. In this case, the participants were able to continue exercising without fatiguing.

But here's the best part of the experiment: The participants increased their fat-burning by 43 percent, compared with controls.

A similar benefit was observed in the second study. In this experiment, ten men who had supplemented with Endurox® experienced a 30 percent increase in fat-burning.

If these studies are any indication, ciwujia-containing supplements may confer a fat-burning advantage. Tapping into fat stores first during exercise, rather than carbohydrates, could definitely help you develop a leaner, trimmer physique.

How to Use It: The recommended adult dose, according to PacificHealth Laboratories (the manufacturer of Endurox®), is two 400 mg caplets taken once a day, 1 to 2 hours before your workout. The company also advises taking it every day, even if you don't exercise daily.

Safety Considerations: PacificHealth Laboratories says its product is safe and has no reported side effects. Clearly, this natural product seems to work best in conjunction with regular exercise. It's definitely worth a try if you're active and want to accelerate your fat-burning potential.

HMB (Beta-Hydroxy Beta-Methylbutyrate)

What It Is: Found in grapefruit, cauliflower, red meat, catfish, and other foods, HMB is a breakdown product of the amino acid leucine. Your body produces it naturally from proteins containing leucine. Since its introduction in 1995, the supplement form of HMB has received a lot of press in some fitness magazines for its presumed fat-burning and muscle-building benefits.

How It Works: Scientists believe HMB prevents muscle breakdown and aids in fat metabolism. Many animal studies have been conducted on HMB, and most have shown that supplementation does two things: It increases lean tissue, and it enhances the immune system. These findings have prompted the use of HMB as an additive in animal feed.

But what about people? There have been a few studies published in scientific journals on the effects of HMB supplementation in humans. At the University of Iowa, researchers conducted two related studies on HMB. In the first, forty-one men were given 1.5 or 3 grams of HMB, or a placebo, daily while participating in a strength-training program 3 days a week. By the end of 3 weeks, the HMB-takers had gained 63 percent more strength than the others. Plus, muscle breakdown during exercise was minimized among the HMB-supplemented group.

In the second study, twenty-eight volunteers took either 3 grams of HMB or a placebo, and strength-trained 6 days a week for 7 weeks. By the end of the study period, the HMB-takers had lost twice as much body fat as those taking the placebo.

In another study, female athletes who took 3 grams of HMB daily boosted their strength by 7 percent, compared with a placebo-supplemented group.

HMB may increase endurance, too. In one experiment, cyclists increased their performance and training intensities dramatically while supplementing with HMB for 2 weeks.

Based on this collection of studies, HMB appears to increase muscle mass and strength, prevent muscle breakdown, support fat loss, and possibly boost stamina. The research certainly gives high marks to HMB, and I think you'll see a lot more studies on HMB in the future.

Other Benefits: In the area of AIDS research, a growing number of studies show that malnourished HIV-infected patients may develop the disease more quickly, primarily because of muscle-wasting (cachexia). To help prevent this, some researchers are experimenting with HMB combined with other amino acids. Their goal: to see whether the mixture will slow down muscle-wasting. The mixture is believed to supply immune cells with the amino acids they need so that muscle stores won't be depleted, and to retard muscle breakdown with HMB supplementation. The approach makes sense in theory, but results are not yet conclusive.

How to Take It: HMB is possibly worth a try, especially if you're a serious, hard-training bodybuilder or weight lifter. What kind of results can you expect? The world's leading authority on HMB, Dr. Steve Nissen, was quoted in the magazine *Muscle Media* as saying that if you strength-train and typically gain 2 pounds of muscle every few weeks, you can possibly gain 3 or 4 pounds of muscle while on HMB.

The recommended dosage is 3 grams daily, taken in divided doses, three times a day. One of those doses should be a few hours before your workout, to give the supplement time to peak in your system and help maximize strength and muscle gains. Additionally, researchers speculate that HMB may work well with carnitine to encourage fat loss.

As for diet, it's best to consume adequate protein while supplementing with HMB and working out with weights—about 1 gram of protein per pound of body weight. Protein supplies the construction material (amino acids) for muscle growth and repair.

Safety Considerations: HMB could ultimately turn out to be a bona fide natural alternative to dangerous steroids for athletes who desire to build muscle. But further testing is needed to determine the safety of HMB, particularly if taken in large doses.

Meal-Replacement Diet Aids

What They Are: Available as bars, in cans, or as mix-it-yourself powders, meal-replacement diet aids, also called "meal replacers," are formulated to reproduce as closely as possible the nutrition you would get from food, complete with carbohydrates, protein, fat, fiber, vitamins, minerals, and other natural ingredients.

How They Work: Meal replacements were originally developed to feed patients in hospitals and nursing homes (where they are still used), but are now marketed for general use. Manufacturers recommend replacing a meal or two with their products to help you shed pounds—or using them as healthful between-meal snacks.

But how well do they work?

Presented at the 1997 annual meeting of the American Society of Clinical Nutrition, a study from the University of Ulm in Germany found that a meal-replacement diet can help take pounds off—and even keep them off. One hundred people participated in the study and were divided into two groups. The first group followed a prescribed low-fat meal plan that consisted of 1,500 calories a day. The second group consumed the same amount of calories, obtained through one low-fat meal a day and two meal replacements of 220 calories each. The diets were followed for 12 weeks.

All the participants completed the program. The dieters in the meal-replacement group lost an average of 17 pounds—significantly more than those who followed the low-fat meal plan.

The researchers followed up with the dieters after two years to see how well they had kept their weight off. The dieters who had lost weight by using meal replacements maintained their losses much more successfully than those on the prescribed meal plan. The researchers concluded that using meal replacements as part of a diet program is an effective way to lose way and keep it off for at least 2 years.

But another study begs to differ. According to a poll of 95,000 readers of *Consumer Reports*, 24 percent of the readers who had tried liquid meal-replacement diets gave them low marks. The readers' major complaints included an average loss of just 3 to 4 percent of their weight; feelings of hunger; and weight regain as soon as they stopped using the diet aid.

What's more, other studies suggest that if you eat meal replacements at breakfast and lunch, you're more likely to binge-eat on real food at dinner—undoing any calorie-cutting good achieved earlier in the day.

How to Use Them Wisely: The safest and best use of meal replacements is as a supplement to your diet rather than as a substitute for meals. Occasional use, when you're going to miss a meal, is fine, and then you might want to drink two at a time, rather than one. Meal replacements are also great supplements for athletes and exercisers, who typically require a higher-caloric diet, and are an excellent way to add calories and nutrients to the diet without adding much bulk.

To help shed pounds, use meal replacements as a midmorning or midafternoon snack. Eating five times a day (three main meals and two snack meals) encourages fat loss. That's because every time you eat a meal, your metabolic rate goes up. As part of digestion and absorption, heat is given off, and this elevates your metabolic rate. So if you eat meals throughout the day, your metabolism is constantly charged up. Meal replacements can help you squeeze in those extra meals.

You can buy meal replacers in health food stores, gyms, sporting goods stores, pharmacies, and grocery stores. The bar and canned versions are a bit pricey—up to $2 a serving. You can save money using the powder form, although the powders take more time to fix.

Bars and canned meal replacers, however, are very convenient to pack. But since the canned versions don't taste good warm, try freezing the can overnight and let it thaw in your gym bag, briefcase, or purse the next day. It will be cold enough to enjoy when you're ready to drink it.

Safety Considerations: When eaten as a healthy snack, meal replacements are a supersafe choice—one of the best snacks around. Only when they are used as part of a restrictive diet are there potential problems. In other words, the products are safe; it's their misuse in dieting that is often unsafe.

Using them on a regular basis to replace a couple of meals a day is walking a nutritional tightrope. You're severely restricting food, and possibly skimping on vital nutrients. Plus, such regimens are hard to stick to for very long. You soon cave in to food urges and eventually regain your weight, plus more. Furthermore, some of these products are very high in sugar (which contributes to fat gain).

Additionally, a few studies have found that people who follow very low-calorie diets (1,000 calories or less), including meal-replacement diets, may develop gallstones, a problem that affects one in ten people. Formed in the gallbladder, gallstones are crystal-like structures that may be as small as a grain of sand or as large as a golf ball.

In a study published in the *International Journal of Obesity Related Metabolic Disorders*, forty-seven obese women followed a 925-calorie-a-day diet consisting of four daily servings of a liquid meal replacement, plus one prepackaged dinner meal. The diet lasted for 26 weeks.

By week 17, six of the dieters had developed gallstones. One of them eventually required a cholecystectomy (gallbladder removal). Those who suffered from gallstones had a number of factors in common: a greater rate of weight loss, higher triglycerides, and higher cholesterol. (Most gallstones are composed primarily of crystallized cholesterol.) While the study did not attempt to explain the relationship between low-calorie dieting and the formation of gallstones, the researchers noted that dieters on meal-replacement diets should be checked for gallstones.

The message in all this: Meal replacements have an important place in nutrition—especially if you lead an on-the-go lifestyle and need a quick, convenient, healthy snack—but they are not always best used to substitute for meals on an ongoing basis.

CHOOSING A HEALTHY
MEAL-REPLACEMENT FORMULA

· Look for a product that approximates the macronutrient profile of a healthy diet—roughly 65 percent carbohydrates, 20 percent protein, and 15 percent fat.

· Find a product that is low in refined sugar. If the first two or three ingredients on the label are sugar, corn syrup, or fructose, the product is probably high in sugar, which can contribute to obesity. The carbohydrate source should be a rapidly digestible form, either a sucrose/glucose combination or glucose polymers.

· If you are lactose-intolerant (unable to digest milk properly), look for a product that is lactose-free.

· Select a product that has a lower fat content. A plus to having some fat in these products is taste. Fat improves the palatability of meal replacements, subduing any "vitamin-like" aftertaste. Some meal replacers are promoted as having a higher fat content—around 30 percent or more. There's no advantage in this, however.

· As for micronutrients, there is little need to purchase a meal replacement with vitamins and minerals in excess of the recommended daily requirements. You'll only be wasting your money. Meal replacements are not supposed to be vitamin or mineral pills, but supplements that provide extra calories.

· Watch out for meal replacements that hype unproven ingredients such as boron, vanadium, or herbs as energy boosters. Some herbs do provide an energy lift, but it comes from the caffeine they contain. One of the best natural additives is creatine, which provides an extra source of muscle energy, particularly when combined with carbohydrates. (See chapter 9.)

BEST LEFT ALONE

Grapefruit Diet Pills

What They Are: First popularized in Hollywood in the 1930s and again in the 1980s, the grapefruit diet is back, reincarnated in pill form. Grapefruit diet pills contain a grapefruit extract (often the insoluble fiber pectin) along with other herbs, fibers, or vitamins. The ingredients vary from product to product. (There is a supplement called grapefruit seed extract. It's not intended for fat loss, though, but is supposed to be a good anti-fungal remedy.)

What They Do: Grapefruit diet pills have been promoted to burn off fat or cellulite, either by following a very-low-calorie diet (roughly 800 calories) or by eating as much as you want—depending upon the dietary recommendations that accompany the pills. There is no valid scientific evidence supporting these claims. Eating lots of grapefruit daily or popping several grapefruit pills a day will not help you lose weight. The small amount of pectin you ingest from these pills is better obtained by eating real grapefruits, oranges, and other citrus fruits.

Safety Considerations: By itself, the grapefruit pectin in these pills is not harmful. However, some of these products are formulated with undesirable ingredients such as phenylpropanoline. You must check labels.

Vanadyl Sulfate

What It Is: The supplement vanadyl sulfate is a commercial derivative of vanadium, a trace mineral found in vegetables and fish. The body needs very little vanadium, and more than 90 percent of what is taken in is excreted in the urine. To the knowledge of the medical community, no one has ever been diagnosed with a vanadium deficiency disease.

What It Does: As a supplement, vanadyl sulfate is supposed to have a tissue-building effect by moving glucose and amino acids into the muscles faster and elevating insulin to promote growth. But the evidence for this has been found only in rats. Still, vanadyl sulfate is being aggressively marketed as a tissue-building supplement for strength trainers and athletes. It is also an ingredient in many natural weight-loss supplements, usually in tiny amounts.

But does it work the magic its promoters say it does? A group of researchers in New Zealand asked the same question. In a 12-week study, forty strength-trainers (thirty men and ten women) took either a placebo or a daily dose of vanadyl sulfate in amounts matched to their weight. So that strength could be assessed, the strength-trainers performed bench presses and leg extensions in one- and ten-repetition sets during the course of the experiment.

The study found that vanadyl sulfate did not increase lean body mass. There were some modest improvements in strength-training performance, but these improvements were short-lived, tapering off after the first month of the study. About 20 percent of the strength-trainers felt extremely tired during and after training.

Safety Considerations: Experts at the USDA Human Nutrition Research Center in Grand Forks, North Dakota, where the most authoritative work on vanadium has been conducted, say there's no reason for anyone to supplement with this mineral, even if you have trouble metabolizing glucose. At high doses, vanadium is extremely toxic and may cause excessive fatigue. But it's probably not harmful in the small amounts you find in some natural diet products.

DHEA (Dehydroepiandrosterone)

What It Is: DHEA is a steroid naturally secreted by the adrenal glands. In fact, it is the most abundant steroid in the bloodstream, concentrated mostly in brain tissues. The body's natural production of DHEA steadily declines after age 30.

DHEA is readily available as a supplement, sold in pharmacies, grocery stores, health food stores, and department stores. Some of these supplements come in the form of wild yam extracts that claim DHEA activity and potency but, in fact, have neither.

Near-magical properties have been attached to DHEA, ranging from increased sex drive to higher energy levels. Bodybuilders, strength-trainers, athletes, and exercisers take it with the hope that it will build muscle and burn fat.

How It Works: DHEA breaks down and is converted to both estrogen and testosterone in the body. (A word of warning: An excess of these sex hormones has been linked to a greater risk of prostate and breast cancers—so it may be beneficial, and for a good reason, that DHEA falls off naturally with age.)

Still, the fact that DHEA turns into testosterone, a muscle-building steroid, makes it very appealing to bodybuilders and other athletes who want to pack on muscle. But there's no real evidence to support a muscle-building effect.

Most of the research on DHEA supplementation has been conducted on animals. However, there have been a number of human experiments, too. Some of these have centered on weight loss, but with mixed results. One thing is clear, however: DHEA seems to encourage weight loss in men, but not in women.

Safety Considerations: The National Institute on Aging (NIA) has warned consumers that there is insufficient proof that DHEA is beneficial, and that it may produce such side effects as confusion, headaches, drowsiness, and liver damage, as well as breast and prostate cancers. Additionally, the NIA feels that DHEA should be available by prescription only—a conviction shared by the FDA. It is unwise to tinker with your body's hormonal system unless you are under close medical supervision. Any potential benefits of DHEA supplementation are far outweighed by its risks.

Over-the-Counter Diet Pills

What They Are: Not to be confused with natural weight-loss supplements, these pills contain a drug, an amphetamine derivative called phenylpropanolamine (PPA). PPA is approved by the FDA as an over-the-counter weight-loss aid. It is also present in many nasal decongestants, cough syrups, and cold remedies.

How They Work: The drug in these pills is a mild stimulant. It acts on the central nervous to speed up the heart rate. However, as a stimulant, it is weaker than ephedrine. PPA curbs hunger, presumably by acting on the brain to suppress appetite. It also causes a release of the hormone noradrenaline (norepinephrine), which liberates fatty acids from storage.

Many studies conducted on PPA support its ability to suppress the appetite. It is less effective at encouraging actual weight loss, however. One study found that volunteers lost only 2 pounds in 6 weeks while using PPA.

Safety Considerations: There is controversy over the risk to healthy people who take PPA. Some studies indicate that even in normal doses it can raise blood pressure in people with normal readings; and there are many reports of other side effects, including headaches, nervousness, and anxiety.

A dangerous irony exists in the availability of this drug. It may indeed help overweight people; however, they are the ones most likely to suffer from high blood pressure, heart disease, thyroid disease, or diabetes—conditions that make the use of PPA medically inadvisable.

There is great potential for abuse of PPA diet products, particularly among young users. The U.S. Public Health Service has noted that young people, ages 10 to 29 years, account for 40 percent of all the PPA-related problems reported to poison control centers. This is troubling, since some people, especially teenagers, can suffer stroke if they exceed the recommended dosage (50 to 75 mg daily). One case, reported in *The Journal of Pediatrics*, described a 17-year-old girl who suffered a stroke following a suicide attempt involving an overdose of five diet aid pills (a total of 375 mg of phenylpropanolamine).

In 1991, a team of researchers reviewed 142 cases of adverse drug reactions to PPA and over-the-counter products containing it. Among their findings: twenty-four cases of brain hemorrhaging, eight cases of seizures, and eight deaths—all associated with PPA use.

This drug should not be taken with any other PPA-containing medication. Nor should it be taken with any agent containing ephedrine or other stimulants. PPA also interacts dangerously with certain anti-depressants, such as monoamine oxidase inhibitors (MASs). The combination can cause life-threatening complications. Anyone with an illness or disease should consult a doctor before taking PPA.

FIFTEEN

YOUR PERSONAL FAT-FIGHTING STRATEGY

With hundreds of natural weight-loss supplements lining the shelves of health food stores and pharmacies, it's easy to feel overwhelmed. As you survey the throng of pills and potions, you might begin to wonder: Which one should I buy?

The first step is to give some thought to your personal weight-loss situation. Analyze your goals: Do you need to curb your appetite, tweak your metabolism, gain more energy, or destress your life to counter emotional overeating?

Next, look through the following profiles. See where you fit in, and what the supplement recommendations are. Once you've identified your niche, follow the guidelines, and you'll be well on your way to a shapelier body.

Many natural weight-loss supplements can be used concurrently, but be careful about taking a handful of different products at the same time. It's unclear how well some combinations work. They may enhance the effects of each other; they may not.

It's better to try one supplement or product at a time. Give it several weeks before deciding whether it's helping you lose weight. If you stop seeing results from one that works, "cycle" it; that is, go on and off the supplement. Take it for a couple weeks, discontinue it, and then resume supplementation. Remember, too, that what works for someone else may not work as well for you. Each of us is quite different, not only in the way we look and act but also in how our bodies respond to different nutrients. The chart at the end of this chapter provides a snapshot look at how to use various natural weight-loss supplements.

Your personal fat-fighting strategy must include diet and exercise. After identifying which supplements you might need, be sure to read appendix A and appendix B, on planning a diet and an exercise program.

YOU'RE OVERWEIGHT AND WANT TO BURN OFF EXTRA POUNDS

You're committed to changing your diet and becoming more active. But you want to give your body a little shove on its way to trimness.

Natural fat-fighters such as pyruvate, carnitine, chromium, lipotropics, and possibly CLA are your best bets. Pyruvate is sometimes formulated with chromium, so there is probably no problem taking these two together. Likewise, chromium is often found in lipotropic and carnitine supplements. To avoid megadosing on chromium, it's best not to take a chromium-containing pyruvate supplement and a chromium-containing lipotropic at the same time.

Supplements containing fat-binding fibers, such as chitosan, should not be combined with other natural weight-loss supplements, since fibers may usher other nutrients from the body. Some studies suggest that excessive fiber in the diet decreases the absorption of calcium, iron, zinc, and other minerals. That's why it's advisable to take your fiber supplements alone; they should not be taken at the same time you take your multivitamin/mineral supplement.

YOU'RE AN OVEREATER, WITH AN OUT-OF-CONTROL APPETITE

If you're ravenous a good deal of the time and overindulging is your downfall, then natural appetite suppressants should be your first line of defense. Hydroxycitric acid (HCA) has a good track record, so you may want to try it first. 5-HTP has a little less research behind it, but shows promise. You may want to check out an amino acid combination supplement such as PhenCal, since it has been tested by its manufacturer with good results. But don't take HCA, 5-HTP, and an amino acid combo all at the same time. Try one at a time, to avoid any unexpected side effects.

HCA and pyruvate supplements can be taken concurrently—to fight fat and your appetite at the same time. But if you experience any unusual reaction, discontinue one or the other, or both.

YOU'RE AN EXERCISER WHO WANTS TO VITALIZE, ENERGIZE—AND BURN MORE FAT

An excellent supplement in your case is MCT oil. Because MCT oil is a food fat, it can be used in conjunction with other natural weight-loss supplements. No restrictions apply (unless you have a medical condition that would preclude its use). The beauty of MCT oil is that you can use the low-carbohydrate strategy (a proven dietary fat-burner) by replacing some of your carbs with the oil, and not feel the corresponding dip in energy levels. (Chapter 8 explains how to do this.)

Is your goal to build fat-burning muscle? With the help of a nutritious diet and a strength-training program, creatine supplementation is a must. Creatine is generally compatible with other nutritional supplements.

Pyruvate is an excellent choice, too, since it increases the glycogen in your muscles, builds endurance, and encourages the body to burn fat before carbohydrates. It appears that pyruvate can be taken safely with most sports and weight-loss products, including MCT oil and creatine.

You may also want to try a product containing ciwujia (see chapter 14), which may encourage greater fat usage during exercise. No information on its compatibility or interaction with creatine or other supplements exists. Until more is known, it is probably advisable to take ciwujia by itself.

YOU'RE AN EMOTIONAL EATER WHO BINGES UNDER STRESS

To calm the storms of emotional overeating, try a temporary regimen of St. John's wort or kava kava. Sometimes these herbs are combined in a single product. There's not much information on whether they are compatible with other natural weight-loss supplements, so it is prudent to take these herbs alone while you attempt to destress your life. Once you have a period of calm eating under your belt, discontinue them and switch to another natural weight-loss supplement.

YOU'RE A MAINTAINER WHO WANTS
TO KEEP LOST WEIGHT OFF

Nearly 95 percent of those who go on diets and lose weight regain that weight, plus interest, within five years. So the real key is keeping weight off. No one supplement will help you do that, although pyruvate taken in maintenance doses is believed to help somewhat.

Success or failure at keeping weight off ultimately depends on multiple factors. Among them are fat intake, diet, and exercise patterns. In an intriguing study, a group of dietitians explored just what makes people take off weight and keep it off. They surveyed people who had participated in a worksite weight-control program at a Midwestern university campus between 1987 and 1990. This particular program was behaviorally oriented and lasted six months each time it was offered. The dieters met once a week for an hour for the first 6 to 8 weeks, and then twice a month for the rest of the 6 months. Fourteen men and fifteen women participated in the study.

Information from the dieters was taken 6 months and 42 months after completing the program. The dieters completed questionnaires on their diet; weight loss and regain patterns; exercise habits; and social support from spouse, children, friends, and coworkers. Measurements such as weight and height were taken as well.

Some interesting findings emerged from both follow-ups: Twenty of the dieters had regained weight. Of significance was that these regainers had a chronic history of yo-yo dieting (going on and off diets, bouncing up and down in weight). The regainers ate more of their calories at dinner than the maintainers did. And the nine dieters who had maintained their weight tended to eat less total fat. They also exercised more and for longer periods of time.

In another fascinating study of maintainers, formerly obese men and women who had kept their weight off for more than five years said that a "trigger" event had prompted them to shed pounds permanently. Trigger events included medical problems such as low back pain, constant fatigue, or varicose veins; emotional trauma in which a wife lost her husband because she was too fat; and appearance issues in which someone became disgusted after seeing his or her body in a photograph.

On average, the maintainers had cut their fat intake to under 30 percent of their diet, ate five meals daily, and exercised regularly. Most lost between 66 and 100 pounds, and were able to maintain an average loss of 30 pounds. This was a very large study, with 629 women and 155 men participating.

Both studies provide important clues on how to keep pounds off. Here are some tips.

- Keep your fat intake low—about 15 to 20 percent of total daily calories.

- Eat your heaviest meals earlier in the day. There's a better chance they'll be burned off by exercise and other activities. Big evening meals tend to be metabolized when you're sleeping—a time when calories can turn into fat more easily.

- Eat frequently throughout the day. Eating at least five meals daily has a stimulating effect on your metabolism—just what you need to keep your body's fat-burning wheels in motion.

- Exercise regularly, choosing an activity you enjoy.

- If you're a yo-yo dieter, get your mind off dieting for a while. Instead, put your energy into becoming more active.

NOW IT'S UP TO YOU

There is a natural feel-good ecstasy associated with a fit body—and you can experience it! Decide today that you're no longer going to live in an overburdened body, but in one that moves, breathes, and lives in healthy liberty.

As you begin to commit to a fitter lifestyle, try not to look at diet, supplementation, and exercise as chores to be endured, but as challenges that will take your body to new levels of health and fitness. Natural weight-loss supplements can help you on your journey, along with a good diet and exercise you enjoy.

Once you reach your destination, just think what you'll gain: a leaner, fitter figure; more energy and greater stamina; sounder sleep; improved general health; greater confidence; less stress and anxiety; a better outlook on life; and more.

Who wouldn't want all that?

Now . . . go for it!

FAT-FIGHTING STRATEGIES

SUPPLEMENT	OVERWEIGHT	OVEREATER	EXERCISER	EMOTIONAL EATER	MAINTAINER
Pyruvate	Pyruvate is reputed to help with fat-loss by encouraging the body to burn fat preferentially. 4 to 6 g daily.	Pyruvate can be taken with natural appetite suppressants and to encourage weight loss. 4 to 6 g daily.	Pyruvate may build more glycogen in your muscles so that you can work out more intensely for greater fat-burning. 4 to 6 g daily.		About 2 g daily of pyruvate is recommended for maintaining a weight loss.
Carnitine	Supplemental carnitine may aid in fat-metabolism. 1,000 to 1,200 mg daily.	Carnitine can be taken with natural appetite suppressants. 1,000 to 1,200 mg daily.	Research shows carnitine may help liberate more fatty acids during exercise, for greater endurance. 1,000 to 1,200 mg daily.		A daily supplement of carnitine (1,000 to 1,200 mg) may help your body utilize fat better, as well as protect your heart.
Chromium	Supplementing with chromium may assist fat-metabolism. 200 mcg daily.	Chromium may help moderate cravings by keeping blood sugar levels normalized. 200 mcg daily.	Supplementing with chromium may help your body build muscle. 200 mcg daily.		The recommended daily dose of chromium is 50 mcg to 200 mcg.
Lipotropics	Lipotropics provide nutritional insurance against fatty buildup in the liver. Follow manufacturer's dosage instructions.		Endurance or aerobic-type exercisers may benefit from additional choline.		

FAT-FIGHTING STRATEGIES (continued)

SUPPLEMENT	OVERWEIGHT	OVEREATER	EXERCISER	EMOTIONAL EATER	MAINTAINER
Fibers	Fat-binding fibers such as chitosan may decrease fat-absorption and storage.	Fat-binding fibers such as psyllium are a healthful addition to any diet to normalize elimination.	Follow a high-fiber diet for good health. 20 to 35 grams daily.	Follow a high-fiber diet for good health. 20 to 35 grams daily.	Follow a high-fiber diet for good health. 20 to 35 grams daily.
HCA	HCA is reputed to have some fat-fighting benefits. 500 mg daily, 3 times daily before meals.	HCA may help suppress your appetite. 500 mg daily, 3 times daily before meals.		HCA may help suppress your appetite. 500 mg daily, 3 times daily before meals.	
5-HTP		5-HTP helps suppress the appetite, though not as powerfully as some natural agents. 50 mg to 100 mg daily.			
Amino Acids		Certain amino acid formulations appear to curb appetite.			
MCT Oil	A good supplement to use with a low-carb diet, 1 to 3 tablespoons daily.		Exercisers often combine MCT oil with carbs to help extend endurance.		A good all-around supplement to use in the diet. 1 to 2 tablespoons daily in a maintenance program, to replace some of the conventional fats in your diet.

SUPPLEMENT	OVERWEIGHT	OVEREATER	EXERCISER	EMOTIONAL EATER	MAINTAINER
Creatine			Creatine is beneficial for building strength and workout intensity, indirectly affecting fat-burning. 10 to 25 g daily for loading, depending on your weight.		Take 2 to 5 g daily for maintenance if you're an exerciser.
Guggul	Guggul is reputed to aid in fat-metabolism.				
St. John's Wort				St. John's wort may provide natural relief for depression and the tendency to overeat that accompanies it in some people. Follow dosages on label.	
Kava Kava				Kava kava may provide natural relief for stress and anxiety, and the tendency to overeat that accompanies it in some people. Follow dosages on label.	

FAT-FIGHTING STRATEGIES (*continued*)

SUPPLEMENT	OVERWEIGHT	OVEREATER	EXERCISER	EMOTIONAL EATER	MAINTAINER
CLA	Preliminary studies support a fat-loss benefit. 2.5 to 5 g daily.				
HMB			HMB reputedly increases strength and reduces body fat in athletes and exercisers. 3 g daily.		
Ciwujia			Ciwujia appears to encourage the body to burn fat stores preferentially over carbs during exercise. 400 mg twice daily.		
Meal Replacers	Use as a snack or to replace no more than one meal a day. Discontinue if replacing a meal leads to hunger and cravings.	May help curb appetite when used as a between-meal snack.	Meal replacers can be taken before a workout to boost energy or afterward to initiate muscle recovery and growth.		Occasional use to replace a meal or use as a convenient snack may assist in weight control.

A 21-DAY EATING PLAN

Without question, natural weight-loss supplements work most effectively in combination with the right diet and a regular exercise program. Below, you'll find a nutritious diet plan based on the U.S. Department of Agriculture's dietary guidelines, which help ensure that you obtain maximum nutrition from your meals.

Featuring 21 days of menus, this plan shows you how to design meals for maximum nutrition. It is not a rigid diet, but a general guide for how to eat each day. You may want to follow this plan exactly as written, or adapt it to your own food preferences.

On average, the plan provides approximately 1,500 calories a day; usually no more than 25 percent of those calories comes from fat—which is the fat consumption ceiling recommended by health authorities. Active men may want to increase calories to 2,000 or more daily. This can be accomplished by eating larger servings of grains and breads, vegetables, and fruits.

This diet is moderately high in protein and provides moderate amounts of carbohydrates—two dietary strategies that encourage fat loss.

Many people are not sure how much weight they should lose. Loss of only 5 to 10 percent of body weight may improve many of the problems associated with overweight, such as high blood pressure and diabetes. If you are trying to lose weight, do so slowly and steadily. A generally safe rate is 1/2 to 1 pound a week until you reach your goal. Avoid crash weight-loss diets that severely restrict calories or the variety of foods.

DAY 1

Breakfast

1 poached egg
1/2 cup All-Bran cereal

1 cup skim milk
1/2 grapefruit

Midmorning Snack

1 medium apple

Lunch

> Quick-fix fajita: 2 corn tortillas, 6 tablespoons black beans (cooked),
>   2 tablespoons chopped onions, 2 tablespoons chopped green pepper,
>   2 tablespoons salsa
> 1 tomato, sliced
> 1/2 cup cooked brown rice
> 1/2 cup fruit salad, water-packed

Midafternoon Snack

> 1 cup nonfat yogurt with 1 tablespoon low-sugar strawberry preserves

Dinner

> 4 ounces chicken breast, baked
>   (skin removed)
> Caesar salad: 2 cups shredded romaine lettuce, 6 tablespoons raw
>   shredded carrot, 6 tablespoons raw chopped cucumber, 1 tablespoon
>   regular Caesar salad dressing

Daily calories: 1360; 26 percent of calories from protein, 62 percent from
carbohydrates, 12 percent from fat; 39 grams of fiber.

DAY 2

Breakfast

> Banana soyshake: Blend one frozen banana, 1 cup soy milk, 1 tablespoon
>   honey

Midmorning Snack

> 1 cup fruit-flavored nonfat or low-fat yogurt

Lunch

> Tuna salad: 3 ounces tuna (water-packed), 2 cups leaf lettuce, 1 tomato
>   (chopped), 3 tablespoons *low-calorie* French dressing
> 1 medium boiled potato
> 3 dried figs
> 1 cup skim milk

Midafternoon snack

> 8 Triscuit crackers   2 ounces fat-free cheddar cheese

Dinner

    4 ounces lean broiled round steak
    1 cup cooked broccoli
    1/2 cup cooked beets

Daily calories: 1,509; 32 percent of calories from protein, 55 percent from carbohydrates, 13 percent from fat; 28 grams of fiber.

DAY 3

Breakfast

    1 cup nonfat yogurt   1/2 cup grapefruit juice
    2 ounces granola cereal

Midmorning Snack

    2 low-sodium rice cakes   2 ounces firm tofu

Lunch

    Gourmet sandwich: 2 slices enriched French bread, 2 ounces goat cheese,
        1 cup leaf lettuce, 1 tablespoon *low-calorie* Italian salad dressing
    1 cup fresh strawberries (or other fruit in season)

Midafternoon Snack

    2 fresh apricots

Dinner

    3 ounces grilled salmon   1 cup cooked mixed vegetables
    1/2 cup brown rice

Daily calories: 1,508; 24 percent of calories from protein, 50 percent from carbohydrates, 26 percent from fat; 20 grams of fiber.

DAY 4

Breakfast

    1 cup liquid egg substitute, scrambled
    1 cup cooked oatmeal
    1 cup skim milk
    1 cup fresh strawberries (or other fruit in season)

Midmorning Snack

    1 cup fruit salad (water-packed)

Lunch at a Fast-Food Restaurant

    Chef's salad   8 ounces 1 percent low-fat milk

Midafternoon Snack

    1 raw carrot (chopped) and 1/2 green pepper (chopped) with 2 table-
       spoons green onion dip

Dinner

    4 ounces turkey breast, baked   1 medium baked potato
    1/2 cup coleslaw

Daily calories: 1,327; 35 percent of calories from protein, 43 percent from
carbohydrates, 22 percent from fat; 21 grams of fiber

DAY 5

Breakfast

    1 poached egg   1/2 cup orange juice
    1 toasted English muffin

Midmorning Snack

    1 cup plain nonfat yogurt, sweetened with 1 tablespoon honey
    1 medium apple

Lunch

    Tuna pita sandwich: 3 ounces tuna (water-packed), 1 cup alfalfa sprouts,
       1 tomato (sliced), 2 tablespoons low-calorie mayonnaise, 1 pita bread
    1 fresh peach
    1 cup skim milk

Midafternoon Snack

    1 cup carrot juice   2 low-sodium rice cakes

Dinner

> 1 cup vegetarian chili
> Caesar salad: 2 cups romaine lettuce, 1/2 small onion (chopped), 1/2
>   green pepper (chopped), 1 tablespoon regular Caesar salad dressing

Daily calories: 1,554; 23 percent from protein, 62 percent from carbohydrates, 15 percent from fat; 41 grams of fiber.

DAY 6

Breakfast

> 1 cup oat bran (cooked), sprinkled with 2 tablespoons toasted wheat germ
> 1 banana
> 1 cup skim milk

Midmorning Snack

> 8 ounces nutritional energy drink

Lunch

> Chicken salad: 3 ounces chicken breast, 1 cup leaf lettuce, 2 tablespoons
>   low-fat mayonnaise, 1 sliced tomato
> 6 dried apricot halves

Midafternoon Snack

> 3 cups plain popcorn

Dinner at a Restaurant

> 4 ounces grilled swordfish
> 1 medium baked potato
> Salad: 2 cups leaf lettuce, 1 green pepper (chopped), 1/2 cup raw shred-
>   ded carrot, 1/4 cup chopped onion, 2 tablespoons regular French
>   dressing

Daily calories: 1,620; 26 percent of calories from protein, 55 percent from carbohydrates, 19 percent from fat; 22 grams of fiber.

DAY 7

Breakfast

> Tofu colada: Blend together 2 ounces silken tofu, 1/2 cup crushed pineapple in its own juice, 1/2 frozen banana, 1 cup skim milk, 1/2 teaspoon coconut extract

Midmorning Snack

> 1 cup plain nonfat yogurt
> 1 cup fresh raspberries (or other fruit in season)

Lunch

> 1 cup lentil soup   1/2 cup coleslaw
> 1 whole wheat roll

Midafternoon Snack

> 1 medium orange

Dinner

> 4 ounces turkey breast, baked   1 cup cooked brussels sprouts
> 1 medium sweet potato   1 tablespoon margarine

Daily calories: 1,340; 26 percent of calories from protein, 60 percent from carbohydrates, 14 percent from fat; 43 grams of fiber.

DAY 8

Breakfast

> 1 cup liquid egg substitute, scrambled
> 1/2 cup Bran Buds cereal
> 1 cup skim milk
> 1/2 grapefruit

Midmorning Snack

> 1 cup fruit-flavored nonfat or low-fat yogurt

Lunch

> Mediterranean sandwich: 1/2 cup garbanzo beans (pureed and mixed
> with 1 tablespoon olive oil), 1 cup leaf lettuce, 1 tomato (sliced).
> Place all ingredients in one pita pocket.
> 1/2 cup fruit salad (water-packed)

Midafternoon Snack

> 1 medium apple

Dinner

> 4 ounces round steak, grilled or broiled
> 1 ear of corn
> 1 cup cooked broccoli

Daily calories: 1,614; 28 percent of calories from protein, 58 percent from
carbohydrates, 14 percent from fat; 41 grams of fiber.

DAY 9

Breakfast

> Healthy French toast: Beat 1 large egg with 1/2 cup skim milk. Dip 2
> slices enriched cracked wheat bread in mixture, and brown them in a
> skillet that has been coated with vegetable spray. Serve with 2 table-
> spoons light syrup.
> 1 fresh peach

Midmorning Snack

> Fruit shake: Blend 1 cup frozen raspberries with 1 cup plain nonfat yogurt

Lunch

> Tuna salad: 3 ounces tuna (water-packed), 2 cups leaf lettuce, 1 tomato
> (chopped), 1/4 cup onions (chopped), 3 tablespoons *low-calorie* French
> dressing
> 1 medium boiled potato

Midafternoon Snack

> Sports nutrition bar

Dinner

> 4 ounces chicken breast, baked or grilled
> 1/2 cup butternut squash
> 1 cup green beans

Daily calories: 1,598; 28 percent of calories from protein, 58 percent from carbohydrates, 14 percent from fat; 25 grams of fiber.

DAY 10

Breakfast

> Scrambled egg whites (4)   1 cup strawberries
> 1 granola bar   1 cup skim milk

Midmorning Snack

> 8 ounces nutritional energy drink

Lunch

> Roast beef sandwich: 3 ounces sliced lean roast beef, 1 cup leaf lettuce,
>   1 tablespoon low-fat mayonnaise, 2 slices enriched cracked wheat
>   bread
> 1 tomato (sliced)
> 1 cup grapes

Midafternoon Snack

> 2 low-sodium rice cakes   1 medium apple

Dinner

> 4 ounces baked ocean perch   1/2 cup cooked corn
> 1 cup cooked kale

Daily calories: 1,561; 25 percent of calories from protein, 50 percent from carbohydrates, 25 percent from fat; 20 grams of fiber.

DAY 11

Breakfast

> 1 cup Cracklin Oat Bran cereal   1 banana
> 1 cup soy milk

Midmorning Snack

    1 cup fruit-flavored nonfat or low-fat yogurt

Lunch

    Spinach salad: 2 cups fresh chopped spinach, 2 chopped hard-boiled
        eggs, 1/4 cup chopped onion, 1/2 cup chopped fresh mushrooms,
        3 tablespoons *low-fat* French dressing
    1 bran muffin

Midafternoon Snack

    1 medium apple

Dinner

    4 ounces low-fat baked ham   1 cup cooked brussels sprouts
    1 medium sweet potato

Daily calories: 1,553; 20 percent of calories from protein, 60 percent from
carbohydrates, 20 percent from fat; 29 grams of fiber.

DAY 12

Breakfast

    Egg white omelet: Combine 1 tablespoon minced onion, 1 tablespoon
        minced green pepper, 1 tablespoon fresh tomato bits, 1 ounce grated
        fat-free cheddar cheese, 1 slice low-fat ham (cut into bits), and 4 egg
        whites. Mix well. Pour into pan that has been coated with vegetable
        spray and cook omelet until done.
    1 bran muffin
    1/2 cup grapefruit juice

Midmorning Snack

    1 cup nonfat yogurt with 1 tablespoon low-sugar strawberry preserves

Lunch at a Fast-Food Restaurant

    Taco salad

Midafternoon Snack

    1 fresh peach

Dinner

> Italian vegetables: In a pan coated with vegetable spray, cook together
> until tender 1 cup eggplant (peeled and cubed), 1 cup zucchini,
> 4 ounces canned mushrooms (drained), and 1/2 onion (chopped).
> Top with 1/2 cup low-calorie spaghetti sauce and non-fat Parmesan
> cheese.
> 1/2 cup spinach or whole wheat pasta

Daily calories: 1,563; 25 percent of calories from protein, 50 percent from
carbohydrates, 25 percent from fat; 27 grams of fiber.

DAY 13

Breakfast

> Yogurt orangeras: Blend together 1/2 cup plain nonfat yogurt, 1/2 cup
> orange juice, 1/2 cup frozen raspberries, and 1 tablespoon honey.
> 2 granola bars

Midmorning Snack

> 1 cup strawberries   1 cup nonfat plain yogurt

Lunch

> Quick-fix fajitas: Combine 1/2 cup heated low-fat refried beans, 1 tomato
> (chopped), and 2 tablespoons jalapeno peppers in two heated flour
> tortillas.

Midafternoon Snack

> 1 medium apple

Dinner at a Steakhouse

> 6 ounces rib eye steak
> 1/2 cup cooked broccoli
> Salad: 2 cups leaf lettuce, 1/2 cup shredded carrots, 1/2 cup chopped
> green pepper, several cucumber slices, 3 tablespoons *low-fat* Italian
> dressing

Daily calories: 1,531; 24 percent of calories from protein, 54 percent from
carbohydrates, 22 percent from fat; 27 grams of fiber.

DAY 14

Breakfast

Scrambled egg whites (4)
1 cup cooked oatmeal with 2 tablespoons raisins
1 cup skim milk
1/2 cup grapefruit juice

Midmorning Snack

1 medium apple

Picnic Lunch

2 slices enriched French bread
2 ounces fat-free cheddar cheese
Chopped raw veggies: 1 cup broccoli, 1 cup cauliflower, 1 carrot

Midafternoon Snack

1 cup skim milk   1 bran muffin

Dinner

4 ounces turkey breast, baked   1/2 cup peas
1/2 cup mashed sweet potatoes   1 cup melon balls

Daily calories: 1,480; 30 percent of calories from protein, 60 percent from carbohydrates, 10 percent from fat; 28 grams of fiber.

DAY 15

Breakfast

Peachy protein shake: Blend vanilla-flavored nutritional energy drink with
    1 cup frozen peaches.
1 cup cooked oatmeal

Midmorning Snack

1 cup carrot juice   1 medium apple

Lunch

Tuna salad: 3 ounces tuna (water-packed), 2 cups leaf lettuce, 1 tomato
(chopped), 3 tablespoons *low-calorie* French dressing
1 bran muffin

Midafternoon Snack

4 whole wheat crackers
6 tablespoons fat-free cottage cheese

Dinner

1 cup vegetarian chili   1/2 cup coleslaw

Daily calories: 1,383; 23 percent of calories from protein, 67 percent from
carbohydrates, 10 percent from fat; 52 grams of fiber.

DAY 16

Breakfast

1 cup nonfat yogurt mixed with 1 cup low-fat granola
1/2 cup orange juice

Midmorning Snack

1 pear

Lunch

Egg salad pita: Mix 2 hard-boiled eggs with 1 tablespoon low-calorie
mayonnaise and 1 teaspoon yellow prepared mustard. Place in pita
bread pocket with 1 cup sprouts (or lettuce).
1 cup raw broccoli

Midafternoon Snack

1 cup skim milk   1 cup fruit salad

Dinner

4 ounces haddock, broiled or baked
1 cup asparagus spears

Daily calories: 1,433; 25 percent of calories from protein, 56 percent from
carbohydrates, 19 percent from fat; 20 grams of fiber.

DAY 17

Breakfast

> 1 cup Cracklin Oat Bran cereal
> 1 cup soy milk
> 1 cup fresh blueberries (or other fruit in season)

Midmorning Snack

> 1 medium apple   1 cup plain nonfat yogurt

Fast-Food Lunch

> Chicken breast sandwich

Midafternoon Snack

> Sports nutrition bar

Dinner

> 1 cup lentil soup
> Caesar salad: 2 cups shredded romaine lettuce, 6 tablespoons raw
>   shredded carrot, 6 tablespoons raw chopped cucumber, 1 tablespoon
>   regular Caesar salad dressing

Daily calories: 1,601; 19 percent of calories from protein, 55 percent from
carbohydrates, 26 percent from fat; 37 grams of fiber.

DAY 18

Breakfast

> 1 cup egg substitute, scrambled   1 cup skim milk
> 1/2 cup of Cream of Wheat cereal   1 cup melon balls

Midmorning Snack

> 1 medium orange

Lunch

> Ham sandwich: 2 slices low-fat ham, 1 ounce low-fat Swiss cheese, several
>   leaves of lettuce, 1 tablespoon brown mustard, 2 slices light rye bread
> 1 cup chopped cauliflower

Midafternoon Snack

Nutritional energy drink

Dinner at a Fast-Food Restaurant

Chicken salad with 3 tablespoons *low calorie* French dressing

Daily calories: 1,222; 31 percent of calories from protein, 47 percent from carbohydrates, 22 percent from fat; 14 grams of fiber.

DAY 19

Breakfast

1 cup cooked oat bran sprinkled with 2 tablespoons toasted wheat germ
1 banana
1 cup skim milk

Midmorning Snack

3 tablespoons dry sunflower seeds   1 packet raisins (.5 oz)

Lunch

Spinach salad: 2 ounces cubed firm tofu, 2 cups fresh chopped spinach,
    1/4 cup chopped onion, 1/2 cup chopped fresh mushrooms,
    3 tablespoons *low-fat* Italian dressing
1 bran muffin
1 medium apple

Midafternoon Snack

Sports nutrition bar   1 cup skim milk

Dinner

4 ounces chicken breast (skin removed), baked or grilled
1/2 cup green beans
1/2 cup cooked carrots

Daily calories: 1,535; 26 percent of calories from protein, 53 percent from carbohydrates, 21 percent from fat; 26 grams of fiber.

DAY 20

Breakfast

> Healthy French toast: beat 1 large egg with 1/2 cup skim milk. Dip
> 2 slices enriched cracked wheat bread in mixture and brown them
> in a skillet that has been coated with vegetable spray. Serve with
> 2 tablespoons light pancake syrup.
> 1 banana

Midmorning Snack

> 1 cup fruit-flavored nonfat or low-fat yogurt

Lunch

> 1 cup vegetarian chili
> 1 cup fresh raspberries with 1/2 cup skim milk

Midafternoon Snack

> 8 Triscuit crackers   2 ounces fat-free cheddar cheese

Dinner at a Seafood Restaurant

> 4 ounces grilled or steamed shrimp
> 1 cup coleslaw

Daily calories: 1,405; 26 percent of calories from protein, 61 percent from
carbohydrates, 13 percent from fat; 36 grams of fiber.

DAY 21

Breakfast

> Egg white omelet: Combine 1 tablespoon minced onion, 1 tablespoon
> minced green pepper, 1 tablespoon fresh tomato bits, 1 ounce grated
> fat-free cheddar cheese, 1 slice low-fat ham (cut into bits), and 4 egg
> whites. Mix well. Pour into pan that has been coated with vegetable
> spray and cook omelet until done.
> 1 slice enriched cracked wheat toast
> 1/2 cup grapefruit juice

Midmorning Snack

> 1 cup fruit-flavored nonfat or low-fat yogurt

Lunch

> 3 ounces chicken breast (skin removed), baked or broiled
> 1/2 cup homemade carrot-raisin salad
> 1 bran muffin

Midafternoon Snack

> Strawberry shake: Blend until smooth 1 cup skim milk, 1 cup strawberries, and 1 tablespoon honey.

Dinner

> 4-ounce extra-lean hamburger patty, broiled or grilled
> 1 cup stewed tomatoes
> 1/2 cup cooked corn

Daily calories: 1,530; 29 percent of calories from protein, 50 percent from carbohydrates, 21 percent from fat; 22 grams of fiber.

NOTES: For additional information on diet and nutrition, consult two diet books I coauthored: *Lean Bodies: The Revolutionary Way to Lose Body Fat by Increasing Calories* (Summit Publishing Group) and *Power Eating* (Human Kinetics). Both are available in paperback.

Nutrients in the Twenty-One-Day Eating Plan were analyzed using Diet Expert software.

PROPER NUTRITION WHILE DIETING

If you follow an eating plan such as the one above, you will be well-nourished, since the menus generally meet or exceed the recommended daily allowances (RDAs) for certain nutrients. The RDAs are only estimates of the levels of nutrients required by most Americans. Under certain conditions—stress, illness, malnutrition, exercise—we may require a much higher intake of certain nutrients. In fact, many experts contend that the RDAs in their present form are too low for some groups of people. Here's a closer look at several key nutrients provided in this plan.

Antioxidants

Antioxidants such as vitamin C, beta carotene, vitamin E, and selenium are of great interest to scientists because of their potentially beneficial role in reducing the risk of cancer and other chronic diseases. On average, this diet provides a variety of antioxidant nutrients. Still, it is a good idea to supplement daily with an antioxidant multivitamin/mineral formula.

Sodium

Sodium, found mostly in salt, has an important role in the regulation of fluids and blood pressure. However, most people eat more sodium than is needed—an average of 2 to 3 teaspoons of salt every day. A healthier sodium target is 500 mg (the minimum requirement) to 2,400 mg per day. The Twenty-One-Day Eating Plan provides an average of 1,700 mg daily. For perspective, in household measures, a level teaspoon of salt provides about 2,300 milligrams of sodium.

Potassium

Potassium, found in a wide variety of vegetables and fruits, may help reduce the risk of high blood pressure, among other benefits. The minimum requirement for potassium is 1,600–2,000 mg daily; active people may need more (at least 3,500 mg) because potassium can be lost in sweat. The menus on this plan meet or exceed requirements.

Calcium

Many women need to eat more calcium-rich foods to obtain the calcium needed for healthy bones throughout life. Your daily calcium intake should be 1,200 mg (women) or 800 mg (men). Postmenopausal women need about 1,500 mg daily, and women who are pregnant or nursing require between 1,200 and 1,400 mg each day. The eating plan provides approximately 1,400 mg a day of calcium. If you need more, consider taking a supplement, but check with your doctor first.

Iron

Active people and women of childbearing age should eat enough iron-rich foods to keep the body's iron stores at adequate levels. The RDA for adults is 10 mg daily for men and 15 mg daily for women. This food plan provides enough iron to meet daily requirements.

Folate

Folate, also called folic acid, is a B-vitamin that reduces the risk of a serious type of birth defect, helps prevent precancerous changes in the uterus, and may protect against heart disease. The adult RDA for folate is

400 mcg. This plan provides adequate folic acid. Some studies indicate that we may need as much as 800 mcg daily. You may want to supplement with a multivitamin/mineral formula to ensure adequate intake.

Dietary Fiber

To get the protective benefits from fiber, the National Research Council recommends eating 20 to 35 grams of fiber a day. The Twenty-one-Day Eating Plan provides fiber within that range.

EASY FAT-BURNING EXERCISE

The easiest way to shed fat and keep it off is to become more active. Physical activity is an essential part of fat loss, particularly because it increases your metabolism and makes your body more efficient at burning fat.

The more exercise you do, the less you have to worry about calories, and the greater your weight loss will be. By burning 250 to 500 calories a day through exercise, you could lose up to a pound of fat a week (7 x 500 = 3,500)—without restricting food intake. Over a 1-hour period, walking briskly can burn roughly 400 calories; aerobic dancing, about 500 calories; strength-training, 350 calories; gardening, 450 calories, and bike riding, about 250 calories.

By exercising regularly, you're doing your body and your health a huge favor. Years of research show that regular exercise can reduce the risk of heart disease, cancer, diabetes, osteoporosis, obesity, depression, and many other physical and mental ailments.

The key to improving health and fitness lies in getting a minimum of 30 minutes of exercise on most days of the week—a recommendation that's easier than you might think. Here are some ways you can fit in just enough exercise—and make it worthwhile:

- Pursue recreational activities for fun, including biking, hiking, swimming, in-line skating, or any team or individual sports you enjoy.

- Engage in day-to-day lifestyle activities such as gardening, mowing the lawn (on foot), raking leaves, carrying groceries, or walking longer distances to destinations while on errands.

- Devote less time to sedentary activities. Spend more time in activities like walking to the store or around the block. Use stairs rather than elevators. Less sedentary activity and more vigorous activity may help you reduce body fat and disease risk.

· For the best fat-burning results, perform structured activities such as walking, running, jogging, aerobic exercise (in a class), and working out on stationary aerobic equipment, as well as strength-developing exercise sessions.

If you pursue more structured exercise activities, there are ways you can jump-start the fat-burning effect of exercise. If you lift weights, for example, perform some aerobic activity afterward. You'll burn more fat. Here's why: lifting weights uses muscle glycogen for fuel. If your exercise session is long—say, 30 to 45 minutes or more—you can deplete a lot of glycogen. Immediately after weight-training, you start the aerobic portion of your workout—but with a glycogen-needy body. Theoretically, your body will be forced to draw on fatty acids sooner for energy during the aerobics. You'll burn more fat, and get leaner as a result.

Another fat-burning tip is to perform prebreakfast aerobics. By the time you wake up, your body is low on glycogen. With less glycogen, your body has to get fuel from somewhere, so it theoretically starts mobilizing fatty acids from fat stores. More body fat is burned as a result, and you're quickly on your way to a leaner physique.

EXERCISING SAFELY

To make your exercise experience safe and effective, be sure to follow these general guidelines:

1. Have a physical examination, including a stress test, before beginning any program of exercise.

2. Slowly ease into the exercise to prevent injuries. Follow directions for recommended increases in activity. Every little bit helps. Even small increases add up and prepare you for more activity later.

3. Drink plenty of water before, during, and after exercise to prevent your body from becoming dehydrated.

IF YOU PERFORM ENDURANCE-TYPE EXERCISE

1. Wear comfortable, sturdy footwear and comfortable, loose-fitting clothes that suit the temperature where you exercise.

2. To improve your level of cardiovascular fitness, work out at a pace at which you can still carry on a conversation. This should put you at roughly 60 to 70 percent of your maximum heart rate ("moderate intensity").

3. For longer endurance-type exercise sessions, begin with a warm-up, and finish off with a cool-down. These can consist of 5 minutes of walking, light jogging, or other low-intensity work. Aerobic exercise machines have warm-up and cooldown periods built into the exercise program.

4. Breathe naturally and comfortably while exercising.

5. If you feel lightheaded or dizzy, or experience any untoward reaction, stop exercising immediately and seek medical attention.

IF YOU PERFORM STRENGTH-DEVELOPING EXERCISE

1. Consult a qualified exercise specialist to set up a program for you.

2. Work out with weights or perform calisthenics at least twice a week, on nonconsecutive days.

3. Start with a weight you can lift ten to twelve times (the last two repetitions should feel difficult), and perform two sets of each exercise.

4. As you get stronger, try to increase the poundages in 1-, 2-, or 5-pound increments each exercise session.

5. Perform exercises for all major muscle groups: legs, abdominals, back, shoulders, arms, and chest.

6. Breathe comfortably and naturally as you lift weights. Never hold your breath during an exercise. Doing so will build up dangerous pressure, impeding blood flow to and from your brain, and potentially causing a fainting spell.

7. Proper exercise form is essential. Try to concentrate on the body part you are working, without jerking, bending your back unnecessarily, or swaying your body. Such motion robs the muscles of proper stimulation.

8. Lift weights slowly—about 3 or 4 seconds. Lower them even more slowly. Slow lifting and lowering will protect your joints and properly stimulate your muscles.

9. Wear clothing that allows your limbs a full range of motion and is appropriate for the temperature in the gym.

10. Consider working out with a partner as a safety precaution, as well as a motivator.

11. Use safety equipment while strength-training, including collars on dumbbells and barbells, and catch racks on pressing benches and squat racks.

12. If you feel faint or dizzy, or experience any untoward reaction, stop exercising immediately and seek medical attention.

NATURAL WEIGHT-LOSS PRODUCTS

What follows is a list of the major natural weight-loss products on the market, along with their chief ingredients, usage recommendations, and price. It can serve as a handy reference before making any purchases.

PYRUVATE SUPPLEMENTS

Pyruvate Plus™
New Vision International
120 capsules
Two capsules contain 1,200 mg calcium and sodium pyruvate,
3 mg vitamin B_6, 10 mg zinc, 100 mcg chromium, 60 mg cornsilk, 20 mg uva ursi, 10 mg cranberry powder, and 10 mg dihydroxyacetone.
Manufacturer's suggested use: two capsules, two to four times daily, with meals.
Price: from $39.95 to $62.95, depending on discounts available.
Mail order: 1-800-828-6140

Pyruvate Fuel™
Twin Laboratories
30 capsules
Each capsule contains 750 mg calcium pyruvate monohydrate.
Manufacturer's suggested use: three capsules daily, preferably with meals.
Price: $19.95

Pyruvate 500™
Pinnacle
60 tablets
Each tablet contains 500 mg Pyruvate 500™ from calcium and sodium salts of pyruvic acid, plus dihydroxyacetone.
Manufacturer's suggested use: two to four tablets daily, preferably before meals or exercise.
Price: $24.99

Calcium Pyruvate
Natural Balance
90 capsules
Each capsule contains 500 mg pure calcium pyruvate.
Manufacturer's suggested use: six to eight capsules daily, in divided doses.
Price: $27.99

Chroma Slim® (also called Pyruvate-C™)
Richardson Labs
60 caplets
Four caplets contain 2,000 mg calcium pyruvate and 400 mcg chromium picolinate.
Manufacturer's suggested use: two caplets with lunch and dinner, with 8 ounces of water, daily.
Price: $24.99

Pyruvate
Optibolic
60 capsules
Each capsule contains 750 mg calcium pyruvate and 5 mg dihydroxyacetone.
Manufacturer's suggested use: four to six capsules daily.
Price: $32.99

CARNITINE SUPPLEMENTS

GNC L-Carnitine
General Nutrition Corporation
60 capsules
Each capsule contains 500 mg l-carnitine.
Manufacturer's suggested use: one capsule daily.
Price: $39.99

Mega L-Carnitine
Twin Laboratories
60 tablets
Each tablet contains 500 mg l-carnitine.
Manufacturer's suggested use: one tablet daily on an empty stomach, or as directed by a physician.
Price: $36.99

L-Carnitine
Neo Elite Nutrition
60 tablets

Each tablet contains 200 mg l-carnitine.
Manufacturer's suggested use: two tablets three times a day, with meals.
Price: $24.95
Mail Order: 1-800-716-4410; ext 6140

Liquid L-Carnitine 1000
Optimum Nutrition
12 fl. oz.
Two tablespoons provide 1,000 mg l-carnitine and 20 mg vitamin B$_5$ (pantothenic acid).
Manufacturer's suggested use: one serving (2 tablespoons) daily.
Price: $17.99

Acetyl L-Carnitine
Informed Nutrition
30 capsules
Each capsule contains 500 mg acetyl l-carnitine.
Manufacturer's suggested use: one or two capsules daily.
Price: $32.99

LIPOTROPIC SUPPLEMENTS

Nutra Slim
Naturally Fit
60 caplets
Two capsules contain 800 mg milk thistle, uva ursi, choline, dl-methionine, and inositol; 250 mg l-carnitine fumerate; 100 mcg chromium picolinate; 40 mg niacinamide; 10 mg pantothenic acid; 10 mg vitamin B$_6$; and 200 mg panax ginseng, gotu kola, and ginger root.
Manufacturer's suggested use: two tablets with a full glass of water before breakfast and before dinner.
Price: $13.99

Chroma Plus Slim™
Richardson Labs
60 caplets
Four capsules contain 200 mcg chromium picolinate, 500 mg l-carnitine, 2,800 mg lipotropics (choline bitartrate, inositol, and dl-methionine), 200 mg betaine HCL, 99 mg potassium chloride, 10 mg pantothenic acid, and 5 mg vitamin B$_6$.
Manufacturer's suggested use: two caplets with a full glass of water before breakfast and before dinner. To accelerate weight loss, take an additional two caplets before exercising.
Price: $14.99

Advanced Lipotropic Formula™
Parrillo Performance
150 capsules
Each capsule contains 20 mg vitamin B_6, 200 mcg vitamin B_{12}, 25 mg betaine HCl., 200 mcg biotin, 200 mg choline, 50 mcg chromium picolinate, 200 mg inositol, 200 mg l-methionine, 35 mg l-carnitine, and 25 mg pancreatin (an enzyme that helps digest fats and other nutrients).
Manufacturer's suggested use: one capsule with each meal.
Price: $28.00
Mail Order: 1-800-344-3404

System-Six™
Irwin Naturals
60 capsules
Six capsules contain 1,500 mg Citrimax™, 300 mg l-carnitine, lipotropics (100 mg choline bitartrate, 100 mg inositol, 25 mg betaine HCL), 1,125 mcg chromium picolinate, 1,125 mg chromium polynicotinate; herbs (100 mg ginger, 100 mg capsicum, 150 mg green tea extract, 150 mg kola nut extract), 100 mg spirulina, 100 mg trace mineral compound, 20 mg vitamin B_3, 2 mg vitamin B_6, 6 mcg vitamin B_{12}, 1.7 mg vitamin B_2, 30 IU vitamin E, 150 mcg iodine, 400 mcg folic acid, 50 mcg selenium, 60 mg vitamin C, 5,000 IU vitamin A, 300 mcg biotin, and 25 mg potassium.
Manufacturer's suggested use: one or two capsules about 30 minutes before meals three times daily (two capsules for fastest results).
Price: $14.99

Antioxidant Lipoic Acid Formula®
Preventive Nutrition
60 softgels
Two capsules contain 3 mg beta carotene, 200 IU vitamin E, 200 mg vitamin C, 50 mcg selenium, 50 mg alpha-lipoic acid, 10 mg l-glutathione, and 10 mg coenzyme Q-10.
Manufacturer's suggested use: two softgel capsules daily.
Price: $24.99

Alpha-Lipoic Acid
Neo Elite Nutrition
60 capsules
Each capsule contains 100 mg of alpha-lipoic acid.
Manufacturer's suggested use: one capsule two or three times per day with meals.
Price: $19.95
Mail Order: 1-800-716-4410; ext 6140

FAT-BINDING FIBERS

Chitosan
Natural Max
240 caplets
Each caplet contains 250 mg chitosan.
Manufacturer's suggested use: four caps 30 minutes prior to lunch and four more 30 minutes prior to dinner. Always take with 8 ounces of liquid.
Price: $25.99

Biozan-C with Chitosan
Richardson Labs
60 caplets
Four caplets contain 2,500 mg BioZan™ (purified chitosan), betaine HCL, oat bran, aloe, and beta glucan (a nutrient extracted from the cell walls of baker's yeast; it activates immune cells that fight disease and helps lower levels of dangerous cholesterol and triglycerides), and 250 mg chromium picolinate.
Manufacturer's suggested use: two to three caplets with lunch and dinner, with 8 ounces of water, daily. Be sure to drink at least two to four additional glasses of water throughout the day.
Price: $14.99

Chito Trim Chitosan with Thermogenic Formula
Naturally Fit
60 caplets
Four caplets contain 100 mg ChitoMax purified chitosan, 225 mg standardized ma huang (6 percent ephedra), 205 mg green tea, 50 mg yerba maté, 100 mg mustard seed, 400 mg chromium picolinate, 250 mg standardized garcinia cambogia extract, 155 mg hawthorn extract, 85 mg schisandra extract, 150 mg choline bitartrate, and 5 mg vitamin B_6.
Manufacturer's suggested use: two caplets with breakfast and lunch, with 8 ounces of water, daily.
Price: $16.99

Chitosan CP400
Naturally Fit
60 caplets
Six caplets contain 3,000 mg Chitomax purified chitosan and 400 mcg chromium picolinate.
Manufacturer's suggested use: two to three caplets with lunch and dinner, with 8 ounces of water, daily.
Price: $14.99

Lipostat™
Dietworks
90 caplets
Each caplet contains Lipostatin,™ a fat-binding complex of oat fiber, citrus pectin, lipase enzyme, marine fiber concentrate, cellulose croscarmellose sodium, stearic acid, silica, dicalcium phosphate, and magnesium stearate.
Manufacturer's suggested use: one caplet half an hour before meals, three times daily, with a full glass of water.
Price: $29.95

NATURAL APPETITE SUPPRESSANTS

Thin-Thin™
Natural Max
30 tablets
Each tablet contains 141 mg calcium carbonate, griffonia extract (guaranteed potency 98 percent), 200 mg 5-HTP, and 270 mg DMAE bitartrate.
Manufacturer's suggested use: one to two tablets daily. Some individuals may need to take tablets with food during the first few days of consumption.
Price: $39.99

PhenCal 106™
Weider
90 tablets
Six tablets contain 30 mg vitamin B_6, 200 mcg chromium picolinate, 2,700 mg dl-phenylalanine, 300 mg tyrosine, 150 mg l-glutamine, 15 mg 5-HTP, and 60 mg l-carnitine.
Manufacturer's suggested use: two tablets 20 to 30 minutes before each meal, on an empty stomach, with water or juice.
Price: $14.97

MCT OIL

CapTri®
Parrillo Performance
32 fl. oz.
Manufacturer's suggested use: 1/2 to 1 tablespoon with each meal.
Price: $40.00
Mail Order: 1-800-344-3404

CREATINE

Creatine Fuel
Twin Laboratories
120 capsules
Each capsule contains 700 mg creatine monohydrate.
Manufacturer's suggested use: six capsules daily, three before exercise and three after exercise.
Price: $28.59

Creatine Monohydrate
Parrillo Performance
300 grams
Manufacturer's suggested use: Loading cycle: One 5-gram scoop mixed with water or beverage 4 times daily for one to two weeks. Maintenance cycle: One 5 g scoop mixed with water or beverage 2 times daily.
Price: $29.00
Mail Order: 1-800-344-3404

Creatine Monohydrate
Neo Elite Nutrition
375 grams or 775 grams
Manufacturer's suggested use: As a dietary supplement, take 5 grams (one heaping teaspoon) with a carbohydrate-rich meal or drink, four to six times daily for one week, followed by a maintenance dose of one to two 5-gram servings daily thereafter.
Price: $56.95 (375 grams); $105.95 (775 grams)
Mail Order: 1-800-716-4410; ext 6140

Pure Creatine Monohydrate
Pro Performance
Net weight 2 pounds 3.2 ounces
Manufacturer's suggested use: As a dietary supplement, for creatine maintenance, take one heaping teaspoon (5 grams) daily. Mix with juice, milk, or your favorite sports drink. For creatine loading, take four heaping teaspoons (20 grams) per day; one heaping teaspoon at four-hour intervals. Mix with juice, milk, or your favorite sports drink. Continue this process for four days. Do not exceed the loading level for more than four days in any one month period.
Price: $49.99

HCA

HCA 1000™
Naturally Fit
45 caplets
Two caplets contain 2,000 mg standardized garcinia cambogia extract (supplying 1,000 mg HCA).
Manufacturer's suggested use: Take one caplet before breakfast and one before lunch. For additional appetite control, take one before dinner.
Price: $18.99

Chroma Slim HCA 1000™
Richardson Labs
60 caplets
Two caplets contain 2,000 mg garcinia cambogia extract (1,000 mg HCA).
Manufacturer's suggested use: one caplet before breakfast and one before lunch. For additional appetite control, take one before dinner.
Price: $24.49

Chroma Slim™ Appetite Control Bar
Richardson Labs
One 1.5-oz. bar
One bar contains 1,000 mg Citrimax™ (HCA) and 200 mcg chromium. Each bar provides 181 calories.
Manufacturer's suggested use: Eat 30 to 60 minutes prior to a meal or as a between-meal snack.
Price: 99¢ per bar

CitraLean
Advanced Research Products
30 caplets
Each caplet contains 500 mg Citrimax™ (50 percent standardized HCA), 100 mg gymnema sylvestre powder, 1 mg vanadyl sulfate, and 100 mcg chromium (as picolinate and polynicotinate).
Manufacturer's suggested use: one caplet three times per day, preferably half an hour before meals.
Price: $19.99

SlimCaps®
New Vision International
60 capsules
One capsule contains 200 mcg chromium and 453 mg of a proprietary blend

of garcinia cambogia, guarana powdered extract, Siberian ginseng, Brigham tea (a form of ephedra), yucca, cayenne pepper, cinnamon, papaya, kelp, spray-dried apple cider vinegar, soy lecithin, and an enzyme blend.
Manufacturer's suggested use: one capsule with 10 ounces of pure water 30 minutes before breakfast and before lunch.
Price: $28.95
Mail Order: 1-800-828-6140

SlimCaps Extra®
New Vision International
60 capsules
One capsule contains 1,666 IU vitamin A (100 percent as beta carotene), 200 mcg chromium, 10 mg potassium, and 800 mg of a proprietary blend of garcinia cambogia, guarana powdered extract, l-carnitine, licorice root, cayenne pepper, cinnamon, ginger root, panax ginseng, soy lecithin, peppermint, and an enzyme blend.
Manufacturer's suggested use: one capsule with 10 ounces of pure water 30 minutes before each meal.
Price: $39.95
Mail Order: 1-800-828-6140

HCA
Neo Elite Nutrition
90 capsules
One capsule contains 350 mg of Citrimax™.
Manufacturer's suggested use: three capsules 30 minutes before consuming carbohydrate-containing meals, two or three times daily.
Price: $15.95
Mail Order: 1-800-716-4410; ext 6140

Citrimax™
Optibolic
90 caplets
Each caplet contains 500 mg Citrimax™ and 200 mcg chromium picolinate.
Manufacturer's suggested use: one caplet three times a day, before meals.
Price: $19.99

HERBAL DIET AIDS

ThermoPhen™
Pinnacle
60 captabs

Two captabs contain 150 mg St. John's wort (0.3 percent hypericin), 200 mg citrus aurantium (1.5–3 percent synephrine), 100 mg kava kava (40 percent kavalactones), and 200 mg yerba maté.

Manufacturer's suggested use: two captabs, two to three times a day, half an hour before meals.

Price: $16.79

Synephrinol

Pinnacle

120 captabs

Two captabs contain 200 mg citrus aurantium (providing 3 to 6 mg synephrine), and 100 mg Herbolics Support Complex™ (which includes yerba maté).

Manufacturer's suggested use: one or two captabs daily on an empty stomach, with 8 ounces of water.

Price: $24.99

Diet Fuel®

Twin Laboratories

60 capsules

Three capsules contain 335 mg ma huang extract (standardized for 20 mg ephedra alkaloids), 909 mg guarana extract (standardized for 22 percent caffeine), 500 mg garcinia cambogia extract, 200 mcg chromium picolinate, 100 mg l-carnitine, and 100 mg potassium and magnesium phosphate.

Manufacturer's suggested use: three capsules before breakfast or morning workout, three capsules before afternoon and evening meals. Not to exceed nine capsules daily.

Price: $15.99

Diet Fuel® Fat-Free Diet Bar

Twin Laboratories

One 2.54 oz. bar

One bar is fortified with 100 mg l-carnitine, 200 mcg chromium picolinate, 25 mg choline, 50 mcg molybdenum, 1 mg manganese, and 25 mcg selenium. Each bar contains 180 calories.

Manufacturer's suggested use: meal replacement or nutrient-dense, fat-free snack.

Price: $2.49 per bar

Ultra Diet Pep®

Pep Products

60 tablets

Two tablets contain an herbal blend of guarana, Siberian ginseng, green tea extract, gotu kola, dandelion, ginger, passion flower, kelp, gymnema sylvestre, pullulan (an ingredient reputed to help gymnema sylvestre work better to control cravings for sweets), and fennel, 15 mg vitamin B_6, 6 mcg vitamin B_{12}, 100 mg choline bitartrate, 100 mg inositol, 200 mcg chromium, 100 mg bromelain, and 99 mg potassium.

Manufacturer's suggested use: one tablet with a full glass of water midmorning and one tablet midafternoon if desired.

Price: $10.97

Thermogenic Formula™
Optibolic
60 caplets
Each caplet contains 200 mcg chromium picolinate, 250 mg Citrimax™ (calcium salt of garcinia cambogia extract), 150 mg guarana seed powder (9 mg caffeine), 150 mg yerba maté powder (2 mg caffeine), 100 mg cayenne pepper, 100 mg mustard seed powder, 50 mg uva ursi, 50 mg astragalus root extract, 50 mg licorice root powder, 50 mg ginger root powder, and 50 mg Siberian ginseng root powder.

Manufacturer's suggested use: one caplet per day with a morning or midafternoon meal.

Price: $16.99

PhenSafe
Applied Nutrition
90 capsules
Three capsules contain 300 mg St. John's wort (0.3 percent hypericin), 100 mg l-glutamic acid HCL, 20 mg vitamin B_6, 10 mg niacinamide, 8 mg zinc, 200 mcg folic acid, 125 mcg ChromeMate, 100 mcg vitamin B_{12}, 75 mcg selenium, and 640 mg citrus aurantium, licorice root powder, ginger root powder, cayenne powder, mustard seed powder, green tea extract, and fennel seed powder.

Manufacturer's suggested use: two or three capsules (three for maximum results) before meals, with a large glass of water (up to nine caplets daily).

Price: $13.94

Phen-Free™
Neo Elite Nutrition
120 capsules
Four capsules contain 99 mg caffeine, 300 mg citrus aurantium (standardized to 6 percent synephrine), 100 mg yohimbe, 500 mg cordyceps, 500 mg l-tyrosine, 200 mg St. John's wort (0.3 percent hypericin), and 30 mg cayenne pepper powder.

Manufacturer's suggested use: two to four capsules two or three times a day. For best results, consume one dose 30 minutes before a meal and one dose an hour prior to exercise.
Price: $34.95
Mail order: 1-800-716-4410; ext 6140

Diet-Phen™
Source Naturals
45 tablets
Three tablets contain 900 mg St. John's wort extract (0.3 percent hypericin), 150 mg ma huang (standardized extract 8 percent, yielding 12 mg ephedra alkaloids), 500 mg phenylalanine, 50 mg acetyl l-carnitine, 25 mg niacin, 25 mg vitamin B_6, and 200 mcg chromium (polynicotinate and picolinate).
Manufacturer's suggested use: one to two tablets in the morning half an hour before breakfast and one tablet half an hour before lunch, or as recommended by your physician.
Price: $19.99

Herbal Phen-Fen
HPF L.L.C.
Two tablets contain 650 mg St. John's wort extract (0.3 percent hypericin) and ma huang extract.
Manufacturer's suggested use: two tablets two times per day, half an hour before meals.
Price: $24.99

Nutra Phen
Naturally Fit
60 caplets
Four caplets contain 900 mg St. John's wort (standardized 0.3 percent hypericin), 150 mg standardized ma huang (6 percent ephedra, 9 mg), 135 mg green tea, 30 mg yerba maté, 65 mg mustard seed, 400 mcg chromium picolinate, 130 mg standardized garcinia cambogia (50 percent HCA), 100 mg hawthorn extract, 55 mg schisandra extract, 100 mg choline bitartrate, 3 mg vitamin B_6.
Manufacturer's suggested use: two caplets with breakfast and two caplets with lunch. Do not exceed four caplets daily.
Price: $23.95

Therma Lean
Naturally Fit
60 caplets

Two caplets contain 225 mg standardized ma huang (6 percent ephedra), 205 mg green tea, 50 mg yerba maté, 100 mg mustard seed, 200 mcg chromium picolinate, 200 mg standardized garcinia cambogia extract, 155 mg hawthorn extract, 85 mg schisandra extract, 150 mg bitartrate, and 5 mg vitamin B₆.
Manufacturer's suggested use: one caplet with breakfast and one caplet with lunch. Do not exceed two caplets daily.
Price: $17.99

Nutra Lean
Naturally Fit
60 caplets
Two caplets contain 225 mg standardized ma huang (6 percent ephedra), 1,000 mg guarana, 250 mg l-carnitine fumerate, 200 mcg chromium picolinate, 500 mcg vanadyl sulfate, 10 mg alpha-ketoglutarate, and 50 mg medium-chain triglycerides.
Manufacturer's suggested use: two caplets with a full glass of water before breakfast and before lunch. Do not exceed six caplets daily.
Price: $14.99

Gugulipid®
Nature's Fingerprint
90 capsules
Each capsule contains 600 mg commiphora mukul extract granules.
Manufacturer's suggested use: three to five capsules daily, preferably with meals.
Price: $24.99

Kavatrol®
Natrol
30 capsules
Each capsule contains kava root standardized for 30 percent kavalactones in a base of herbs (passion flower, chamomile flower, hops, and schisandra).
Manufacturer's suggested use: one capsule three times per day, preferably before a meal or on an empty stomach.
Price: $12.95

Natural Rest™
Neo Elite Nutrition
60 capsules
Two capsules contain 600 mg kava root standardized for 30 percent kavalactones, 300 mg valerian extract standardized to 0.8 percent valeric acid

(valerian is an herb used to promote sleep and relaxation), and 3 mg melatonin (a natural hormone that appears to help sleep).
Manufacturer's suggested use: two capsules one hour before you go to sleep.
Price: $34.95
Mail order: 1-800-716-4410; ext 6140

St. John's Wort
Nature's Way
100 capsules
Each capsule contains 150 mg of St. John's wort extract with 350 mg of St. John's wort herb, standardized to contain a minimum of 0.3 percent hypericin.
Manufacturer's suggested use: one to two capsules twice a day with water, between meals. For maximum benefit, use for a minimum of two months.
Price: $14.49

St. John's Wort
Neo Elite Nutrition
60 capsules
Each capsule contains 450 mg of St. John's wort standardized to 0.3 percent hypericin.
Manufacturer's suggested use: one capsule two times daily, between meals.
Price: $23.95
Mail order: 1-800-716-4410; ext 6140

Cordyceps 500
Pinnacle
90 tablets
Each tablet contains 500 mg cordyceps in a base of Chinese herbs.
Manufacturer's suggested use: one or two tablets three times a day, with meals and 8 ounces of water.
Price: $39.99

CLA SUPPLEMENTS

Tonalin™ CLA-750
Natrol
30 softgels
Each softgel contains 750 mg CLA, 75 mcg chromium picolinate, 100 mcg capsicum, and 100 mg ginger root.
Manufacturer's suggested use: one to two softgels daily, preferably with low-fat or nonfat milk for maximum protein absorption.
Price: $9.97

Chroma Slim CLA 4000
Richardson Labs
60 caplets
Four caplets contain 4,000 mg CLA.
Manufacturer's suggested use: two caplets with lunch and two caplets with dinner, with 8 ounces of water, daily.
Price: $29.99

Tona-Lean™ 1000 CLA
Action Labs
60 capsules
Each capsule contains 1,000 mg CLA.
Manufacturer's suggested use: one capsule before each meal. Suggested water consumption is eight to ten glasses daily.
Price: $25.99

HMB

HMB
Neo Elite Nutrition
240 capsules
Each capsule contains 250 mg of HMB and 50 mg of potassium phosphate.
Manufacturer's suggested use: four capsules three times daily.
Price: $64.95
Mail order: 1-800-716-4410; ext 6140

CIWUJIA SUPPLEMENTS

Endurox®
PacificHealth Laboratories
60 caplets
Each caplet contains 800 mg ciwujia extract and 130 mg calcium (sulfate).
Manufacturer's suggested use: two caplets once daily (adults).
Price: $14.99

Endurox® Excel™
PacificHealth Laboratories
60 caplets
Each caplet contains 1,200 mg ciwujia extract and 60 IU vitamin E.
Manufacturer's suggested use: two caplets once daily (adults).
Price: $23.95

Time-Release Ciwujia
Optibolics
60 capsules
Each capsule contains 400 mg ciwujia extract and 500 mg Dahluin™ (a carbohydrate).
Manufacturer's suggested use: three to six capsules before working out.
Price: $14.99

Time-Released Ciwujia
Pro Performance
50 capsules
Each capsule contains 250 mg ciwujia extract.
Manufacturer's suggested use: two capsules before extended physical activity.
Price: $11.99

REFERENCES

A portion of the information in this book comes from personal case studies, medical research reports in both popular and scientific publications, professional textbooks and booklets, newspaper articles, audiotapes, Internet data searches, and research abstracts.

INTRODUCTION: LOSING WEIGHT THE NATURAL WAY

Brown, J. 1990. *The science of human nutrition.* San Diego: Harcourt Brace Jovanovich.

C. Everett Koop Foundation. 1995. *Shape Up, America.*

CondoNet. October 1997. The diet pill controversy. Internet web address: www.phys.com.

Connolly, M. 1996. The new (doctor-approved) diet pills. *Good Housekeeping*, June, 141–142.

Editor, *Cancer Weekly*. 1991. Upper-body fat distribution and endometrial cancer risk, 14 October, 26–27.

Editor, *Harvard Health Letter*. 1996. The new diet pills: Fairly (but not completely) safe, 7 (December): 1–2.

Editor, *Journal of the American Dietetic Association*. 1996. Position of the American Dietetic Association: Vitamin and mineral supplementation, 96: 73–77.

Editor, *Prevention*. 1998. Is the new diet pill for you? May, 38, 40.

Evansville Courier. 1996. Nothing's magical, but new fat-fighting drugs show big promise, 10 December, A-9, Evansville, Indiana.

———. 1997a. FDA trying to determine if fen-phen, birth defects linked, 5 October, A-13.

———. 1997b. Users of diet drugs urged to get exam, 14 November, A-23.

———. 1997c. New diet drug with risk factor ok'd, 25 November, A-1.

———. 1998a. Thinner is better, study concludes, 1 January, A-13.

———. 1998b. Hunger hormone believed found, 20 February, A-2.

———. 1998c. Brief use not seen as dangerous, 1 April, C-16.

Federal Trade Commission. 1997a. FTC announces "operation waistline"—a law enforcement and consumer education effort designed to stop misleading weight loss claims, 25 March. Internet web address: www.ftc.gov.

———. 1997b. Advertising cases involving weight loss products and services 1927–April 1997. Internet web address: www.ftc.gov/opa/9703/dietcase.htm.

Fraser, L. 1996. The new diet drugs: They really do help some people lose weight. *Health*, July–August, 52–53.

———. 1997. The diet pill dilemma. *Eating Well*, September, 72–76.

Griffith, H.W. 1988. *Complete guide to vitamins, minerals & supplements*. Tucson, AZ: Fisher Books.

Langer, S. 1990. Fight obesity with dietary therapies. *Today's Living*, April, 8–9.

Marchione, M. 1997. Obesity: Virus may be to blame. *Evansville Courier*, 8 April, A-2. Evansville, Indiana.

New study examines demographic and cultural links to obesity, 4 March. Internet web address: www.pslgroup.com.

1997b. Couch potatoes, not French fries, may be to blame for obesity, 25 July. Internet web address: www.plsgroup.com.

1997c. PSL Consulting Group, Inc. An "ecological" approach to the obesity pandemic, 22 August: Internet web address: www.plsgroup.com.

1997d. PSL Consulting Group, Inc. New role for brain receptor in control of body weight, 27 November. Internet web address: www.plsgroup.com.

Reilly, L. 1997. Standardized issue: What "standardized" means to the consumer of herbal products. *Vegetarian Times*, November, 94.

Sizer, F., and Whitney, E. 1997. *Nutrition concepts and controversies*. 7th ed. Belmont, CA: West/Wadsworth.

USA Today. 1998. 3 in 4 Americans are overweight, 2 February. Internet web address: www.usatoday.com.

CHAPTER 1. PYRUVATE: THE BREAKTHROUGH DISCOVERY THAT REVS UP YOUR FAT-BURNING ENGINE

Allen, A. 1997. Redux, fen-phen, serotonin, pyruvate. *Women's Fitness International*, August 42–45.

Brink, W. 1997. Lean machine: Is pyruvate a weight-loss wonder? *Let's Live*, June, 64–66.

Colker, C., Stark, R., Kalman, D., et al. 1997. Pyruvate: New study finds that it can change the shape of your physique. New Vision International product information pamphlet.

Deboer, L.W., Bekx, P.A., Han, L., and Steinke, L. 1993. Pyruvate enhances recovery of rat hearts after ischemia and reperfusion by preventing free radical generation. *American Journal of Physiology* 265: H1571–H1576.

Editor, *Executive Health's Good Health Report*. 1995. Antioxidants save the day from free radicals, November, 1–2.

Halliwell, B. 1994. Free radicals, antioxidants, and human disease: Curiosity, cause, or consequence? *The Lancet* 344: 721–724.

Langer, S. 1997. Antioxidants: Our knights in shining armor. *Better Nutrition*, May, 46–50.

Mahi, J. 1998. Pyruvate: The natural path to weight loss. *Total Health*, February–March, 36–37.

O'Donnell-Tormey, J., Nathan C.F., Lanks, K., et al. 1987. Secretion of pyruvate: An antioxidant defense of mammalian cells. *Journal of Experimental Medicine* 165: 500–514.

Prokop, D. 1997. *Pyruvate: The super strength, stamina and weight-loss supplement*. Pleasant Grove, UT: Woodland Publishing.

Richardson, S. 1994. The war on radicals. *Discover*, July, 27–28.

Roufs, J.B. 1997a. *Pyruvate: A scientific review and practical guide*. Intelligent Nutrition.

———. 1997b. Pyruvate: The answers to your heaviest questions. Audiotape of lecture. Intelligent Nutrition.

Salahudeen, A.K., Clark, E.C., and Nath, K.A. 1991. Hydrogen peroxide-induced renal injury. A protective role for pyruvate in vitro and in vivo. *Journal of Clinical Investigation* 88: 1886–1893.

Scheer, J.F. 1995. Antioxidants: Free radicals' worst enemy. *Better Nutrition*, October, 50–53.

Stanko, R.T., and Arch, J.E. 1996. Inhibition of regain in body weight and fat with addition of 3-carbon compounds to the diet with hyperenergetic refeeding after weight reduction. *International Journal of Obesity Related Metabolic Disorders* 20: 925–930.

Stanko, R.T., Mullick, P., Clarke, M.R., et al. 1994. Pyruvate inhibits growth of mammary adenocarcinoma 13762 in rats. *Cancer Research* 54: 1004–1007.

Stanko, R.T., Reynolds, H.R., Lochar, K.D., and Arch, J.E. 1992. Plasma lipid concentrations in hyperlipidemic patients consuming a high-fat diet supplement with pyruvate for 6 weeks. *American Journal of Clinical Nutrition* 56: 950–954.

Stanko, R.T., Robertson, R.J., Galbreath, R.W., et al. 1990. Enhanced leg exercise endurance with a high-carbohydrate diet and dihydroxyacetone and pyruvate. *Journal of Applied Physiology* 69: 1651–1656.

Stanko, R.T., Robertson, R.J., Spina, R.J., et al. 1990. Enhancement of arm exercise endurance capacity with dihydroxyacetone and pyruvate. *Journal of Applied Physiology* 68: 119–124.

Stanko, R.T., Sekas, G., Isaacson, I.A., et al. 1995. Pyruvate inhibits clofibrate-induced hepatic peroxisomal proliferation and free radical production in rats. *Metabolism* 44: 166–171.

Stanko, R.T., Tietze, D.L., and Arch, J.E. 1992a. Body composition, energy utilization, and nitrogen metabolism with a severely restricted diet supplemented with dihydroxyacetone and pyruvate. *American Journal of Clinical Nutrition* 55: 771–776.

———. 1992b. Body composition, energy utilization, and nitrogen metabolism with a 4.25-MJ/d low energy diet supplemented with pyruvate. *American Journal of Clinical Nutrition* 56: 630–635.

CHAPTER 2. CARNITINE: THE INTERNAL FAT-BURNER FOR SPEEDIER WEIGHT LOSS

Adams, R. 1990. Carnitine: The amino acid with muscle. *Better Nutrition*, September, 16–18.

Challem, J., and Lewin, R. 1993. What's missing from the RDAs? *Natural Health*, January–February, 56–59.

Clarkson, P.M. 1992. Nutritional ergogenic aids: Carnitine. *International Journal of Sports Medicine* 2:185–190.

Coley, C., and Legino, R.L. 1997. Carnitine deficiency. *Exceptional Parent*, June, 45–46.

Colombani, R., Wenk, C., Kunz, I., et al. 1996. Effects of l-carnitine supplementation on physical performance and energy metabolism of endurance-trained athletes: A double-blind crossover field study. *European Journal of Applied Physiology* 73: 434–439.

DeSimone, C., Ferrari, M., Lozzi, A., Meli, D., et al. 1982. Vitamins and immunity: Influence of l-carnitine on the immune system. *Acta Vitamino Enzymol* 4: 135–140.

Dragan, G.I., Vasiliu, A., Georgescu, E., and Eremia, N. 1989. Studies concerning chronic and acute effects of l-carnitine in elite athletes. *Physiologie* 26: 111–129.

Dragan, G.I., Wagner, W., and Ploesteanu, E. 1988. Studies concerning the ergogenic value of protein supply and l-carnitine in elite junior cyclists. *Physiologie* 25: 129–132.

Editor, *The Lancet*. 1990. Carnitine deficiency, 335 (17 March): 631–633.

Editor, *Let's Live Nutrition Insights*. 1997. Do carnitine and caffeine improve performance? October, 23.

Gormley, J.J. 1996. Healthful weight loss includes l-carnitine, chromium and lipotropics. *Better Nutrition*, May, 40.

Harper, P., Wadstrom, C., Backman, L., and Cederblad, G. 1995. Increased liver carnitine content in obese women. *American Journal of Clinical Nutrition* 61: 18–25.

Kaats, G.R., Wide, J.A., Blum, K., et al. 1992. The short-term therapeutic efficacy of treating obesity with a plan of improved nutrition and moderate caloric restriction. *Current Therapeutic Research* 51: 261–274.

Lerner, M. 1997. Carnitine makers get set for growing product demand. *Chemical Market Reporter*, June, 12.

Occhipinti, M. 1998. L-carnitine: The wonder nutrient. Internet web address: www.afpafitness.com/carnit.htm.

Pierpont, M., Dianne, J., Goldenberg, I.F., et al. 1989. Myocardial carnitine in end-stage congestive heart failure. *American Journal of Cardiology* 64: 56–60.

Regitz, V., Shug, A.L., and Fleck, E. 1990. Defective myocardial carnitine metabolism in congestive heart failure secondary to dilated cardiomyopathy and to coronary, hypertensive and valvular heart diseases. *American Journal of Cardiology* 65: 755–760.

Rowley, B. 1997. Acetyl l-carnitine. *Muscle and Fitness*, May, 126–131.

Saltmarsh, N. 1989. Reach your peak. *Today's Living*, January, 15–17.

Vaughn, L. 1984. Discovering the healing powers of carnitine. *Prevention*, October, 50–54.

Watanbe, S., Ajisaka, R., Masuoka, R., et al. 1995. Effects of l- and dl-carnitine on patients with impaired exercise tolerance. *Japanese Heart Journal* 36: 319–331.

CHAPTER 3: CHROMIUM: THE MIRACLE MINERAL THAT FIGHTS FAT GAIN

Campbell, W.W., and Anderson, R.A. 1987. Effects of aerobic exercise and training on the trace minerals chromium, zinc, and copper. *Sports Medicine* 4: 9–18.

Campbell, W.W., Beard, J.L., Joseph, L.L., et al. 1997. Chromium picolinate supplementation and resistive training by older men: Effects on iron status and hematologic indexes. *American Journal of Clinical Nutrition* 66: 944–949.

Challem, J. 1993. How to use nutritional supplements. *Natural Health*, March–April, 88–98.

Clancy, S.P., Clarkson, P.M., DeCheke, M.E., et al. 1994. Effects of chromium picolinate supplementation on body composition, strength, and urinary chromium loss in football players. *International Journal of Sport Nutrition* 4: 142–153.

Clarkson, P.M. 1991. Nutritional ergogenic aids: Chromium, exercise, and muscle mass. *International Journal of Sport Nutrition* 1: 289–293.

Critchfield, T.S., and Burris, A. 1996. What's the story? *Diabetes Forecast*, April 24–26.

Editor, *Better Nutrition*. 1994. For losing extra weight, try chromium picolinate, September, 13.

Editor, *Better Nutrition*. 1995. For a leaner body mass, try chromium picolinate, January, 44.

Editor, *Better Nutrition*. 1996. Weight-loss aids, with dietary changes, help us reach our goal, February, 36–39.

Editor, *Nutrition Health Review*. 1993. Chromium—little known, seldom used, but very essential to health, Spring, 10.

Editor, *Tufts University Diet & Nutrition Letter*. 1996. Chromium picolinate: Nutritional star or flash in the pan? October, 4–6.

Editor, *Tufts University Diet & Nutrition Letter*. 1997. Chromium picolinate's image tarnished, January, 7.

Evans, G.W. 1994. Chromium: Insulin's cohort. *Total Health*, August, 42–43.

Gormley, J.J. 1997. Dietary chromium is safe—and elemental to good health. *Better Nutrition*, March, 18.

Grant, K.E., Chandler, R.M., Castle, A.L., and Ivy, J.L. 1997. Chromium and exercise training: Effect on obese women. *Medicine and Science in Sports and Exercise* 29: 992–998.

Hochwald, I. 1998. Slim pickins. *Natural Remedies*, March–April, 58–63.

Jaros, T. 1996. Is chromium picolinate safe? *Vegetarian Times*, February, 30–31.

Kozlovsky, A.S., Moser, P.B., Resier, S., and Anderson, R.A. 1986. Effects of diets high in simple sugars on urinary chromium losses. *Metabolism* 35: 515–518.

Mestel, R. 1996. Has chromium lost its luster? *Health*, March–April, 56–57.

Murray, F. 1992. Lower cholesterol with niacin-bound chromium. *Better Nutrition*, February, 32–34.

Nielsen, F.H. 1996. Controversial chromium: Does the superstar mineral of the mountebanks receive appropriate attention from clinicians and nutritionists? *Nutrition Today* 31: 226–234.

Passwater, R.A. 1992. *Chromium picolinate: Breakthrough in sports nutrition.* New Canaan, CT: Keats Publishing.

Press, R.I., Geller, J., and Evans, G. 1990. The effect of chromium picolinate on serum cholesterol and apolipoprotein fractions in human subjects. *Western Journal of Medicine* 152: 41–45.

PSL Consulting Group, Inc. 1997. Chromium may help obese people avoid diabetes, June 30. Internet web address: www.pslgroup.com.

Reading, S.A. 1996. Chromium picolinate. *Journal of the Florida Medical Association* 83: 29–31.

Scheer, J.F. 1993. Niacin-bound chromium. *Better Nutrition*, February, 40–41.

Trent, L.K., and Thielding-Cancel, D. 1995. Effects of chromium picolinate on body composition. *Journal of Sports Medicine and Physical Fitness* 35: 273–280.

CHAPTER 4: LIPOTROPICS: FAT-MOBILIZING NUTRIENTS

Benjamin, J., Levine, J., Mendel, F., et al. 1995. Double-blind, placebo-controlled, crossover trial of inositol treatment for panic disorder. *American Journal of Psychiatry* 152: 1084–1086.

Berdanier, C.D. 1992. Is inositol an essential nutrient? *Nutrition Today* 27: 22–26.

Buchanan, C. 1989. Lecithin supplements: A source of help or hype? *Environmental Nutrition*, June, 1–2.

Clouatre, D., and Brink, W. 1997. Alpha lipoic acid for total performance. *Let's Live*, October, 65–67.

Colombo, V.E., Gerber, F., Bronhofer, M., and Floersheim, G.L. 1990. Treatment of brittle fingernails and onychoschizia with biotin: Scanning electron microscopy. *Journal of the American Academy of Dermatology* 23: 1127–1132.

Editor, *Better Nutrition*. 1994. Vitamin B₆, magnesium may help some PMS patients, October, 16.

Editor, *Better Nutrition*. 1996. Alpha-lipoic acid is an antioxidant that prevents free-radical damage, January, 12.

Hughes, L. 1996. Beauty in a pill: Are supplements today's fountain of youth? *Environmental Nutrition*, May, 1–2.

Kanter, M.M. 1994. Antioxidants and other popular ergogenic aids. In *Proceedings of Nutritional Ergogenic Aids*, November 11–12, Chicago.

Leung, L.H. 1995. Pantothenic acid as a weight-reducing agent: Fasting without hunger, weakness and ketosis. *Medical Hypotheses* 44: 403–405.

Levine, J., Barak, Y., Gonzalves, M., et al. 1995. Double-blind, controlled trial of inositol treatment of depression. *American Journal of Psychiatry* 152: 792–794.

Liebman, B. 1990. PMS: Proof or promises? *Nutrition Action Newsletter*, May, 1–3.

Lombard, K.A., and Mock, D.M. 1989. Biotin nutritional status of vegans, lacto-ovovegetarians, and nonvegetarians. *American Journal of Clinical Nutrition* 50: 486–490.

Malesky, G. 1984. Saving lives with biotin. *Prevention*, August, 26–32.

Mazer, E. 1981. Biotin—the little known lifesaver. *Prevention*, July, 97–102.

Murray, F. 1990. Pantothenic acid: Vitamin on the run. *Better Nutrition*, May, 14–15.

Passwater, R.A. 1995. *Lipoic acid: The metabolic antioxidant*. New Canaan, CT: Keats Publishing.

Song, W.O. 1990. Pantothenic acid: How much do we know about this B-complex vitamin? *Nutrition Today* 25: 19–26.

Vaughn, L. 1984. B$_6$: A spectrum of healing. *Prevention*, June, 30.

Wade, C. 1991. Feed your brain, boost your memory. *Health News & Review*, July–August, 1.

CHAPTER 5. FAT-BINDING FIBERS

Arvill, A., and Bodin, L. Effect of short-term ingestion of konjac glucomannan on serum cholesterol in healthy men. *American Journal of Clinical Nutrition* 61: 585–589.

Baker, E. 1989. High energy naturally enriched foods. *Total Health*, October, 23-27.

Best, D. 1989. Processors pursue the perfect nutritional profile. *Prepared Foods*, March, 79–82.

———. 1996. Nutraceuticals: From theory to practice. *Prepared Foods*, June, 53–56.

Editor, *Better Nutrition*. 1994. Dietary fiber helps some to lose weight, October, 34.

Editor, *FDA Consumer*. 1990. Guar gum diet products under investigation, October, 3–4.

Editor, *Nutrition Research Newsletter*. 1991. Benefits of fiber for dieters, February, 17.

Evansville Courier. 1998. Bran Buds gets FDA endorsement, 18 February, C-9.

Hammock, D. 1997. Trick your stomach. *Good Housekeeping*, March, 117–118.

Kalman, D.S. 1998. Analyzing the latest natural weight-loss supplements. *Muscular Development*, July, 96–98, 152–153.

Kalsa, K.P. 1996. Total herbal weight loss. *Let's Live*, December, 62–65.

Kimm, S. 1995. The role of dietary fiber in the development and treatment of childhood obesity. *Pediatrics* 96: 1010–1014.

Langer, S. 1990. Fight obesity with dietary therapies. *Today's Living*, April, 8–9.

ChitoRich™, 1997. The magic pill for weight loss. Internet web address: members.aol/aubsherbs/chitorch.htm.

National Research Council for Health, Meridian, OH. 1998. *Study report: BioZan®*.

Nelson, L.H., and Tucker, L.A. 1996. Diet composition related to body fat in a multivariate study of 203 men. *Journal of the American Dietetic Association* 96: 771–777.

Passaretti, D., Franzoni, M., Comin, U., et al. 1991. Action of glucomannans on complaints in patients affected with chronic constipation: A multicentric clinical evaluation. *Italian Journal of Gastroenterology* 23: 421–425.

Pechter, K. 1985. Fiber helps your body stay well. *Prevention*, September, 50–57.

Scheer, J. 1989. Fabulous fiber helps decrease cholesterol levels. *Today's Living*, November, 12–14.

Vaughn, L. 1984. Getting the most out of the F complex. *Prevention*, September, 48–54.

CHAPTER 6. 5-HTP: THE MOOD BOOSTER THAT HELPS PREVENT WEIGHT GAIN

BioSynergy Health Alternatives. 1997. 5-HTP vs. SSRIs. Internet web address: www.webfactor.com/biosynergy/5htp.htm.

Cangiano, C., Fabrizio, C., Cascino, A., et al. 1992. Eating behavior and adherence to dietary prescriptions in obese subjects treated with 5-hydroxytryptophan. *American Journal of Clinical Nutrition* 56: 863–867.

Clouatre, D. 1997. 5-HTP and the link between mood and food. *Let's Live*, September, 56–59.

Davidson, C. 1998. Listening to 5-HTP. Internet web address: www.west.net/~lifelink/trypto.html.

Farley, D. 1993. Dietary supplements: Making sure hype doesn't overwhelm science. *FDA Consumer*, November, 8–13.

Schechter, S. 1998. The connection between food and mood. Seacoast Natural Foods. Internet web address: www.seacoastvitamins.com/thinthin.html.

South, J. 1997. 5-hydroxytryptophan: The serotonin solution. Vitamin Research Products. Internet web address: www.vrp.com.

CHAPTER 7. AMINO ACID THERAPY: STOP FOOD CRAVINGS

Brown, J. 1990. *The science of human nutrition.* San Diego: Harcourt Brace Jovanovich.

Campbell, S. 1989. Do muscle builders really build muscles? *AFAA's American Fitness,* September–October, 8–9.

Chadwick, M.J., Gregory, D.L., and Wendling, G. 1990. A double-blind amino acids, L-tryptophan and L-tyrosine, and placebo study with cocaine-dependent subjects in an inpatient chemical dependency treatment center. *American Journal of Drug and Alcohol Abuse* 16: 275–286.

Corpas, E., Blackman, M.R., Robertson, R., et al. Oral arginine-lysine does not increase growth hormone or insulin-like growth factor in old men. *Journal of Gerontology* 48: 128–133.

Editor, *Better Nutrition.* 1995. L-tyrosine helps to boost energy, overcome stress, March, 18.

Editor, *Executive Health's Good Health Report.* 1994. Glutamine: The essential non-essential amino acid, July, 1–2.

Elkins, R. *Nature's phen-fen.* Pleasant Grove, UT: Woodland Publishing.

Felig, P. 1984. Very-low-calorie protein diets. *New England Journal of Medicine* 310: 589–591.

Fisher, H. 1987. On the mend with arginine. *Prevention,* October, 98–106.

Griffith, H.W. 1988. *Complete guide to vitamins, minerals & supplements.* Tucson, AZ: Fisher Books.

Isidori, A., Lo Monaco, A., and Cappa, M. 1981. A study of growth hormone release in man after oral administration of amino acids. *Current Medical Research and Opinion* 7: 475–481.

Jacobsen, B.H. 1990. Effect of amino acids on growth hormone release. *Physician and Sportsmedicine* 18: 68.

Lambert, M.I. 1993. Failure of commercial oral amino acid supplements to increase serum growth hormone concentrations in male body-builders. *International Journal of Sport Nutrition* 3: 298–305.

Langer, S. 1992a. The promise of weight loss metabolizers. *Better Nutrition,* August, 14–15.

———. 1992b. Intelligent weight loss. *Better Nutrition,* November, 26–31.

Malesky, G. 1989. Battling disease with the amino factor. *Prevention,* May, 61–65.

Murray, F. 1989. Lysine keeps heart and bones strong. *Today's Living*, November, 22–23.

Poirot, C. 1997. Sales of herbal diet pills rise—as do warnings. *Fort Worth Star-Telegram*, 22 August.

Taylor, D.S. 1989. Amino acids aid in weight control. *Better Nutrition*, May, 10–12.

Tuttle, D. 1997. Glutamine: Athletic benefits times three. *Let's Live*, September, 71–73.

Welbourne, T. 1995. Increased plasma bicarbonate and growth hormone after an oral glutamine load. *American Journal of Clinical Nutrition* 61: 1058–1061.

CHAPTER 8. MCT OIL: KICK-START YOUR METABOLISM WITH THIS "FATLESS" FAT

Dias, V. 1990. Effects of feeding and energy balance in adult humans. *Metabolism* 39: 887–891.

Dulloo, A.G., Fathi, M., Mensi, N., and Girardier, L. 1996. Twenty-four-hour energy expenditure and urinary catecholamines of humans consuming low-to-moderate amounts of medium-chain triglycerides: A dose-response study in a human respiratory chamber. *European Journal of Clinical Nutrition* 50: 152–158.

Editor, *Better Nutrition*. 1993. Good nutrition can help athletes lose weight, 55: 22–23.

Editor, *Environmental Nutrition*. 1995. MCT oil, 8: 7.

Hill, J.O., Peters, J.C., Yang, D., et. al. 1989. Thermogenesis in humans during overfeeding with medium-chain triglycerides. *Metabolism* 38: 641–648.

Roberson, A., and Parrillo, J. 1997. *Medium chain triglycerides in sports*. Cincinnati, OH: Parrillo Performance.

Seaton, T.B., Welle, S.L., Warenko, M.K., and Campbell, R.G. 1986. Thermic effect of medium and long chain triglycerides in man. *American Journal of Clinical Nutrition* 44: 630–634.

Stubbs, R.J., and Harbron, C.G. 1996. Covert manipulation of the ratio of medium- to long-chain triglycerides in isoenergetically dense diets: Effect on food intake in ad libitum feeding men. *International Journal of Eating Disorders* 20: 435–444.

Van Zyl, C. 1996. Effects of medium chain triglyceride ingestion on fuel metabolism and cycling performance. *Journal of Applied Physiology* 80: 2217–2225.

CHAPTER 9. CREATINE: THE ENERGIZER THAT HELPS DEVELOP BODY-SHAPING MUSCLE

Anderson-Parrado, P. 1997. High-intensity activity + creatine supplementation = muscle power. *Better Nutrition*, November, 16–17.

Armsey, T.D., and Green, G. 1997. Nutrition supplements: Science vs hype. *Physician and Sportsmedicine* 25: 76–92.

Bamberger, M. 1998. The magic potion. *Sports Illustrated*, 20 April, 58–65.

Clarkson, P.M. 1996. Nutrition for improved sports performance. *Sports Medicine* 6: 393–401.

Earnest, C.P., Almada, A.L., and Mitchell, T.L. 1996. High-performance capillary electrophoresis—pure creatine monohydrate reduces blood lipids in men and women. *Clinical Science* 91: 113–118.

Editor. 1998. Creatine. Internet web address: www.life-enhancement.com.

Editor, *Let's Live Nutrition Insights*. 1997. Creatine's benefits grow, October, 22.

Editor, *Penn State Sports Medicine Newsletter*. 1994. The promise of creatine supplements, January, 1–3.

Editor, *Sports Illustrated*. 1997. The carbohydrate of the 90s, 28 July, 26–27.

Evansville Courier. 1997a. Muscle builder gets critical reappraisal, 5 October, B-11. Evansville, Indiana.

———. 1997b. Investigation over in wrestler's death, 12 December, C-4.

Green, A.L., Hultman, E., MacDonald, I.A., Sewell, D.A., and Greenhaff, P.L. 1996. Carbohydrate ingestion augments skeletal muscle creatine accumulation during creatine supplementation in humans. *American Journal of Physiology* 271: E821–E826.

Greenhaff, P. 1994. Can creatine loading improve high power performance? Presented at Nutritional Ergogenic Aids Conference sponsored by the Gatorade Sports Institute, November 11–12, Chicago.

Huggins, S. 1996. Energy supplement stirs debate. *NCAA News*, October, 1 and 16.

Kleiner, S.M., and Greenwood-Robinson, M. 1998. *Power eating*. Champaign, IL: Human Kinetics.

MacIntosh, A. 1996. Exercise therapeutics update and commentary. *Townsend Letter for Doctors and Patients*, December, 30–31.

Parrillo, J. 1995. *Creatine: Why has this become a must supplement among bodybuilders?* Cincinnati, OH: Parrillo Performance.

Sahelian, R., and Tuttle, D. 1997. *Creatine: Nature's muscle builder*. Garden City Park, NY: Avery Publishing Group.

Volek, J.S., Kraemer, W.J., Bush, J.A., et al. 1997. Creatine supplementation enhances muscular performance during high-intensity exercise. *Journal of the American Dietetic Association* 97: 765–770.

CHAPTER 10. HCA (HYDROXYCITRIC ACID): CONTROL YOUR APPETITE NATURALLY—AND LOSE FAT, TOO

Cichoke, A.J. 1994. Nature's unique diet ingredient. *Total Health*, August, 12–14.

———. 1995. An interview with the man who wrote the book on HCA. *Total Health*, April, 22–24.

Clouatre, D. 1995a. *Anti-fat nutrients*. San Francisco: Pax.

———. 1995b. Fat-melting fruit: A weight problem answer? *Health News & Review*, Spring, 4.

Editor, *Better Nutrition*. 1995a. Chromium picolinate, HCA help for weight loss, March, 36.

———. 1995b. Weight loss enhanced with chromium and HCA, August, 34–37.

Gormley, J.J. 1996. Energy balance, exercise and weight loss: Where does HCA fit in? *Better Nutrition*, July, 42–43.

Majeed, M., Rosen, R., McCarty, M., et al. 1994. *Citrin®: A revolutionary, herbal approach to weight management*. Burlington, CA: New Editions.

Murray, F. 1995. Hydroxycitric acid: End the yo-yo weight loss game. *Better Nutrition*, February, 42–47.

Sister, D.L. 1995. Fat-fighting herbs can curb craving, hinder weight gain, deplete calories. *Health News & Review*, Summer, 22.

CHAPTER 11. GUGGUL: A FAT-CONQUERING BOTANICAL

Badmaev, V., and Muhammed, M. 1995. Weight loss, the Ayurvedic system. *Total Health*, August, 32–35.

Best Nutrition, Inc. 1998. Guggul. Internet web address: www.bestnutrition. com/guggul.html.

Editor, *Better Nutrition*. 1993. Ancient Ayurveda still effective against many ills, March, 14.

Gormley, J.J. 1996a. Ancient art of balancing digesting, nutrient absorption, and metabolism. *Better Nutrition*, July, 36–37.

———. 1996b. Sticky gum helps "unstick" blood fats and reduces heart disease risk. *Better Nutrition*, December, 24.

———. 1997a. Three Ayurvedic herbs for cardiovascular protection, and more. *Better Nutrition*, February, 34.

———. 1997b. A trio of health concerns is faced by a trio of Ayurvedic herbs. *Better Nutrition*, June, 28.

Kalsa, K.P. 1996. Total herbal weight loss. *Let's Live*, December, 62–65.

McCaleb, R. 1993. Ayurvedic medicine: A balanced approach. *Better Nutrition*, December, 44–47.

———. 1994. Historic herbals of Ayurvedic medicine. *Better Nutrition*, July 52–54.

Nityanand, S., Srivastava, J.S., and Asthana, O.P. 1989. Clinical trials with gugulipid: A new hyperlipidaemic agent. *Journal of the Association of Physicians in India* 37: 323–328.

Thappa, D.M., and Dogra, J. 1994. Nodulocystic acne: Oral gugulipid versus tetracycline. *Journal of Dermatology* 21: 729–731.

Zucker, M., and Khalsa, K. Purkh Singh. 1997. Ayurveda: Ancient medicine for a modern world. *Let's Live*, 34–39.

CHAPTER 12. KAVA KAVA AND ST. JOHN'S WORT: TWO CALMER-DOWNERS

Andersen-Parrado, P. 1998. The road to long-term weight loss may not be short, but it is safe. *Better Nutrition*, January, 22–23.

Carey, B. 1998. The sunshine supplement: Can a humble herb really chase your blues away? *Health*, January–February, 52–54.

Chapman, N. 1998. St. John's wort. *Natural Lifestyle*, Spring, 12–13.

Foster, S. 1997. Kava kava, a gift of calm from the South Pacific. *Better Nutrition*, May, 54–58.

Hawken, C.M. 1997. *St. John's Wort*. Pleasant Grove, UT: Woodland Publishing.

Hochwalk, L. 1996. Natural stress solutions. *Natural Health*, May–June, 68–80.

Kinzler, E., Kromer, J., and Lehmann, E. 1991. Effect of a special kava extract in patients with anxiety-, tension-, and excitement states of non-psychotic genesis. *Arzneimittelforschung* 41: 584–588.

Langer, S. 1997. Break the chain—control stress with optimal nutrition. *Better Nutrition*, December, 24–28.

Linde, K., Ramirez, G., Mulrow, C., et al. 1996. St. John's wort for depression—an overview and meta-analysis of randomised clinical trials. *British Medical Journal* 313: 253–258.

Sahley, B.J., and Birkner, K. 1988. Stress and weight control. *Total Health*, April, 56–59.

Tyler, V.E. 1997. Nature's stress buster. *Prevention*, October, 90–93.

Volz, H.P., and Kieser, M. 1997. Kava kava extract ws 1490 versus placebo in anxiety disorders—a randomized placebo-controlled 25-week outpatient trial. *Pharmacopsychiatry* 30: 1–5.

Walji, H. 1997. *Kava: Nature's relaxant*. Prescott, AZ: Hohm Press.

Warnecke, G. 1991. Psychosomatic dysfunctions in the female climacteric. Clinical effectiveness and tolerance of kava extract ws 1490. *Fortschritte der Medizin* 109: 119–122.

CHAPTER 13. HERBAL WEIGHT LOSS: THE SKINNY ON FORTY-THREE HERBS

Canning, P. 1995. *Exotic supplements*. Vista, CA: Margaret H. Canning.

Challem, J. 1992. Green gold of the future: Discover the many health benefits of spirulina. *Health News & Review*, Spring, p. G.

Clouatre, D. 1997. Sports nutrients and weight-loss aids. *Let's Live*, June, 50–55.

DeStefani, E., Correa, P., Fierro, L., et al. 1991. Black tobacco, mate, and bladder cancer: A case-controlled study from Uruguay. *Cancer* 67: 536–540.

Dodson, M. 1998. Herbs go from "hippy dippy and voodoo" to mainstream. *Evansville Courier*, 2 January, B-11.

Duke, J.A. 1997. *Green pharmacy*. Emmaus, PA: Rodale Press.

Editor, *Better Nutrition*. 1993. Nutrition helps athletes lose fat, not muscle, March, 24–25.

———. 1994. Losing weight requires careful planning, March, 22.

———. 1995. Flax inhibits cancer and lowers cholesterol, April, 12.

Editor, *Environmental Nutrition*. 1994. Herbal teas touted for weight loss: "Quick fix" with hidden dangers, September, 8.

Editor, *Environmental Nutrition*. 1995. Spirulina: Good source of beta-carotene, but no miracle food, December, 7.

———. 1997. Herbal laxative may be at root of a heart problem, July, 3.

Editor, *FDA Consumer*. 1991. Ban of 111 diet ingredients proposed, January–February, 3.

———. 1997. Supplements with plantain may pose danger, FDA warns, September–October, 5.

Editor, *Morbidity and Mortality Weekly Report*. 1994. Anticholinergic poisoning associated with an herbal tea—New York City, 1994, 24 March, 193–195.

Editor, *Total Health*. 1995. "P" is for parsley, April, 52.

Editor, *Women's Day*. 1998. What you should know about herbal phen-fen, 2 February, 36.

Edwards, T.J. 1994. United States botanic garden. *Total Health*, December, 16–17.

Evansville Courier. 1998. Bandwagon boarded by "sex drug" hopefuls, 3 May, E-6.

Flynn, M.E. 1997. What's hot and what's not. *Environmental Nutrition*, January, 1–3.

Food and Drug Administration. 1997. Warning about herbal fen-phen. Internet web address: www.fda.org.

Foster, S. 1995. Lowly wonders: Two powerfully healing herbs you migh have overlooked (dandelion and stinging nettle). *Mother Earth News*, April–May, 18–19.

———. 1996a. Three top herbs that work so you can sleep. *Better Nutrition*, March, 46–49.

———. 1996b. Bundle up with botanicals to boost your immunity. *Better Nutrition*, November, 64–68.

———. 1997a. Two herbs with a heart for health. *Better Nutrition*, April, 56–61.

———. 1997b. Ginseng: The power plant. *Better Nutrition*, June, 48–54.

———. 1997c. Phytomedicine—harnessing the healing power of plants: 5 herbs for the next millennium. *Better Nutrition*, December, 32–35.

Fraser, L. 1996. The dangers of natural diet aids. *Glamour*, March, 62–64.

Gormley, J.J. 1996a. Gymnema sylvestre: Providing new hope for those with diabetes. *Better Nutrition*, April, 42–43.

———. 1996b. For wound healing, silicon-rich horsetail makes good "horse sense." *Better Nutrition*, May, 30.

Grant, A. 1997. Dieter's teas. *Health Gazette*, August, 2.

Griffith, H.W. 1988. *Complete guide to vitamins, minerals & supplements*. Tucson, AZ: Fisher Books.

Heinerman, J. 1992. Helpers and healers from our desert drugstore. *Health News & Reviews*, Spring, p. E.

Hellmich, N. 1997. Herbal diet aid attacked. *USA Today*, 7 October, 1.

Hobbs, C. 1991. Adaptogens: All-purpose herbs. *East–West*, July–August, 54–61.

Howe, M. 1996. The Chinese medicine chest. *Country Living*, September, 46–48.

Hurley, J.B. 1996. A woman's medicine chest: Ten herbs for women's unique needs. *Vegetarian Times*, July, 86–88.

Kalman, D.S. 1998. Analyzing the latest natural weight-loss supplements. *Muscular Development*, June, 96–98, 204–206.

Keller, B.H. 1994. Reins tightened on diet aids, products must now prove their worth. *Environmental Nutrition*, March, 1–3.

Kennedy, B. 1990. Flax for the diet. *Total Health*, April, 27–28.

———. 1993. Disease prevention: Flax seed endorsed by the FDA. *Total Health*, October, 54.

Krampf, L. 1994. Natural help for hypothyroidism: Diet and exercise can ease your pain. *Vegetarian Times*, November, 122–123.

Langer, S. 1993. Weight loss: Stimulate metabolism naturally. *Better Nutrition*, September, 26–31.

———. 1995. Energizers: Moving mind and body. *Better Nutrition*, August, 40–42.

———. 1997. Get recharged with energizing nutrients. *Better Nutrition*, September, 42–46.

Lee, P.A. 1989. Gymnema sylvestre. *Total Health*, December, 31–32.

Light, L. 1997. Herbs for longevity: Botanicals boost vitality and give you more vibrant health. *Vegetarian Times*, February, 84–86.

Marandino, C. 1997. Ephedra falls under FDA jurisdiction. *Vegetarian Times*, September, 18–19.

Mayell, M. 1997. 25 power herbs. *Natural Health*, September–October, 115–132, 164–175.

Mazer, E. 1983. Natural remedies for fluid retention. *Prevention*, December, 106–112.

McCaleb, R. 1992. Ginseng energy booster: This popular ancient herb is used to boost immunity and energy and to increase strength. *Better Nutrition for Today's Living*, January, 34–36.

———. 1997. Straight talk on herbs. *Natural Health*, March–April, 42–44.

———. 1993. Astralagus for immunity. *Better Nutrition*, May, 52–54.

Mindell, E. 1998. *Earl Mindell's supplement bible*. New York: Fireside.

Mowrey, D. 1992. Alfalfa. *Health News & Review*, Winter, 17.

———. 1993. Cascara sagrada: Herbal tonic to get you moving. *Health News & Review*, Summer, 17.

———. 1995. Astragalus: A potent immune booster, effective with colds, flu, cancer. *Health News & Review*, Winter, 18.

———. 1996a. Explore a unified, nutrient-based approach to body fat management. *Better Nutrition*, June, 42–43.

———. 1996b. Using tonic herbs for improved brain function is a smart idea. *Better Nutrition*, December, 28–29.

———. 1997. Valerian root, passion flower, and ginkgo are top "neurtonic" herbs. *Better Nutrition*, January, 34.

Murray, F. 1990. Alfalfa: Nature's digestive aid. *Better Nutrition*, May, 12–13.

Nix, E. 1995. New ways to cope with bloating. *Redbook*, February, 39–40.

Phillips, B. 1998. New study supports fat-loss supplement claims. *Muscle Media*, May, 24–25.

Phillips, C. 1994. A Harvard study: Cranberry juice for women's health. *Total Health, October,* 26.

Pieralisi, G., Ripari, P., and Vecchiet, L. 1991. Effects of a standardized ginseng extract combined with dimethylaminoethanol bitartrate, vitamins, minerals, and trace elements on physical performance during exercise. *Clinical Therapy*, May–June, 337–347.

Ridker, P.M. 1989. Health hazards of unusual herbal teas. *American Family Physician* 39: 53–56.

Scheer, J.P. 1991. Fight cholesterol with alfalfa. *Better Nutrition*, August, 12–14.

Schnirring, L. 1997. Ephedrine safety rules proposed. *Physician and Sportsmedicine* 15: 29.

Stauth, C., Beinfield, H., and Korngold, E. 1994. Gold medal herbs. *Natural Health*, May–June, 84–94.

Tyler, V.E. 1997. Weight-loss herbs. *Nutrition Forum*, May–June, 21.

———. 1998. Nix alfalfa for arthritis. *Prevention*, May, 97.

Webb, G. 1997. Medicine from the sea. *Vegetarian Times*, April, 94–96.

Wiley, C. 1991. The medicinal side of mushrooms: Ancient Eastern remedies for modern Western maladies. *Vegetarian Times*, March, 64–68.

Woolley, B.H. 1991. The latest fads to increase muscle mass and energy: A look at what some athletes are using. *Postgraduate Medicine* 89: 195–204.

Ziegler, J. 1989. A sweet spice for diabetics: Cinnamon may boost the effects of insulin. *American Health*, November, 96–97.

CHAPTER 14. MORE DIET PRODUCTS: WHAT TO TRY, WHAT TO LEAVE ALONE

Armsey, T.D., and Green, G. 1997. Nutrition supplements: Science vs hype. *Physician and Sportsmedicine* 25: 76–92.

Berkowitz, K.F. 1990. Over-the-counter diet pills: Who's minding the store? *Environmental Nutrition*, November, 1–3.

Bilger, B. 1997. A food lover's guide to fats. *Health*, September, 88–95.

Butterworth, D. 1994. Do I need a commercial program? *Vibrant Life*, January–February, 14–16.

Callahan, M. 1997. *DHEA: The miracle hormone*. New York: Penguin Books.

Dilsaver, S.C., Votolato, N.A., and Alessi, N.E. 1989. Complications of phenylpropanolamine. *American Family Physician* 39: 201–206.

Eastern Massachusetts Better Business Bureau. 1995. Weight loss promotions. White paper.

Eder, R. 1997. Drug stores find diet/weight loss and sports nutrition a "natural" fit. *Drug Store News*, 18 August, CP50–CP52.

Editor, *AIDS Weekly Plus*. 1997. Nutrient mixture's ability to prevent muscle wasting in AIDS patients examined, 23 June, 7.

Editor, *American Family Physician*. 1991. Adverse effects of phenylpropano-lamine. 43: 286.

Editor, *American Health*. 1995. Weight loss products, December, 14–15.

Editor, *Better Nutrition*. 1996. Weight-loss aids, with dietary changes, help us reach our goal, February, 36–39.

Editor, *Cancer Weekly Plus*. 1996a. Drinking milk regularly may cut risk of breast cancer, 4 November, 22–23.

———. 1996b. Compounds in milk may reduce early indicators of cancer, 11 November, 8.

Editor, *Child Health*. 1989. Stroke following overdose with a common diet aid and decongestant. June, 4–5.

Editor, *Health Facts*. 1991. Deaths have been reported from ingestion of excessive does of OTC weight loss pills, January, 3.

Editor, *Muscle Media*. 1998. HMB: An interview with Dr. Steve Nissen, April, 120–127.

Editor, *Tufts University Diet & Nutrition Newsletter*. 1985. Grapefruit pills are back, April, 2.

Greene, H. 1997. Comments. Internet web address: www.ftc.gov/bcp/weightloss/greene.htm.

Hearn, W. 1996. New food supplement said to build strength safely. *American Medical News*, August, 40–41.

Kalman, D.S. 1998. Analyzing the latest natural weight loss supplements. *Muscular Development*, July, 96–98, 152–153.

Marandino, C. 1997. Is time running out for longevity supplements? *Vegetarian Times*, October, 20–21.

Nature's Own. 1998. Conjugated linoleic acid. Internet web address: www.naturesownusa.com/CLA.html.

Nissen, S., Sharp, R., Ray, M., et al. 1996. Effect of leucine metabolite beta-hydroxy-beta-methylbutyrate on muscle metabolism during resistance-exercise training. *Journal of Applied Physiology* 81: 2095–2104.

Raloff, J. 1994. This fat may fight cancer several ways. *Science News* 145: 182–183.

Schechter, S. 1997. Fat intake can boost weight loss, if we are selective about our choices. *Better Nutrition*, June, 26.

Scheer, J.F. 1991. Meal replacement formulas: The nutritious diet choice. *Better Nutrition*, April, 12–14.

Sheehy, G. 1997. DHEA: Does it hold the secret of youth? *The Natural Way*, January–February, 38–42.

Spirt, B.A., Graves, L.W., Weinstock, R., et al. 1995. Gallstone formation in obese women treated by a low-calorie diet. *International Journal of Obesity Related Disorders* 19: 593–595.

Walsh, J. 1997. Powerful pills or pricey placebos? A look at sports nutrition supplements. *Environmental Nutrition*, May, 1–2.

INDEX

ABOUT THE AUTHOR

Maggie Greenwood-Robinson, Ph.D., is one of the country's top health and medical authors. She is the author of *21 Days to Better Fitness* and the coauthor of nine other fitness books, including the national bestsellers *Lean Bodies; Lean Bodies, Total Fitness; High Performance Nutrition; Power Eating;* and *50 Workout Secrets.*

Her articles have appeared in *Let's Live, Shape, Women's Sports and Fitness, Working Woman, Muscle and Fitness, Female Bodybuilding and Fitness,* and many other publications. She is a member of the advisory board of *Physical Magazine.* In addition, she has taught body-shaping classes at the University of Southern Indiana. She has a doctorate in nutritional counseling and is a certified nutritional consultant.